Contents

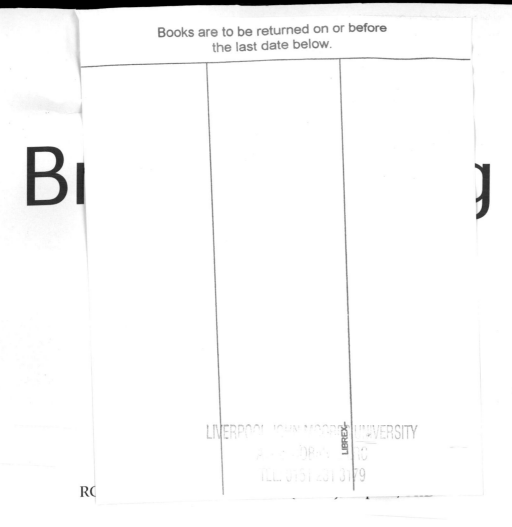

B g

RC

and

Linda Martindale
MA (Hons), MBA, PGCertTHE

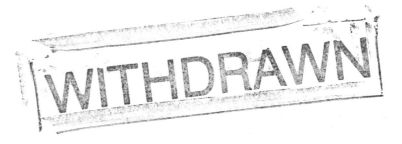
Radcliffe Publishing
New York

Radcliffe Publishing Ltd
18 Marcham Road
Abingdon
Oxon OX14 1AA
United Kingdom

www.radcliffepublishing.com
Electronic catalogue and worldwide online ordering facility.

British Library Cataloguing in Publication Data

A catalogue record for this book is available from the British Library.

ISBN-13: 978 184619 361 3

The paper used for the text pages of this book is FSC certified. FSC (The Forest Stewardship Council) is an international network to promote responsible management of the world's forests.

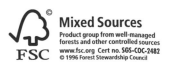

Mixed Sources
Product group from well-managed
forests and other controlled sources
www.fsc.org Cert no. SGS-COC-2482
© 1996 Forest Stewardship Council

Typeset by Pindar NZ, Auckland, New Zealand
Printed and bound by TJI Digital, Padstow, Cornwall, UK

About the authors

Janet Dalzell RGN, RM, BN, MN

Janet has over 20 years of experience working with maternity services, service redesign, and community nursing and public health departments. Her predominant interests during this period have been the promotion, support and protection of breastfeeding throughout these various settings. More recently, she was appointed as the Health Improvement Principal for Breastfeeding in a large NHS board area of Scotland. This role has a specific remit to improve women's experiences during the initiation and continuation of breastfeeding, with a particular focus on women who live in the most disadvantaged areas. This in-depth knowledge and expertise will be shared throughout this text to challenge all practitioners to work to improve service delivery, and lead with a diverse range of women in all social groups and a range of professionals in the UK National Health Service (NHS).

Elizabeth Rogerson RGN(UK), RN(USA), HV, MA (Hons), Dip Ed, PhD

Elizabeth has over 25 years of nursing experience in the UK and the USA, specialising in community and child health. She has a further 20 years of experience as a nurse educator, specialising in the design and development of practice-based learning, delivered by distance learning to an international market. Elizabeth spent 10 years teaching in London as a clinical lecturer. She has held the position of Senior Lecturer and also of Head of the Distance Learning Centre at the University of Dundee, Scotland. She left nursing temporarily to study politics and history as a full-time student at the University of Dundee, Scotland, and achieved an MA (with honours) in politics and history in 1979. Since 1990 her interests have focused on the design, development and delivery of distance learning to support practice-based learning in nursing and the healthcare professions, and she completed a PhD in this area in 2004.

Linda Martindale MA (Hons), MBA, PGCertTHE

Linda is a Lecturer in the School of Nursing and Midwifery, University of Dundee. She specialises in the teaching of research and evidence-based practice, and is currently studying for a PhD in this area. She has a diverse background, having initially completed an MA (Hons) in economics and French at the University of St Andrews, and subsequently completed an MBA at the University of Strathclyde. However, in recent years she has worked exclusively in nursing education, and has developed a particular interest in e-learning and the use of online resources in learning. To this book she also brings the user perspective, having breastfed her own four children and encountered many of the problems as well as the joys of success along the way.

Introduction

ABOUT THIS BOOK

Healthcare professionals and leading healthcare organisations globally are in agreement that, with only a few exceptions, breastfeeding is best for both mother and baby. This view represents a changing tide in healthcare opinion that has taken place over the last 20 years and has been influenced by an accumulating body of research evidence and international policy guidelines, which are making an impact on breastfeeding policy and practice throughout the world.

This book aims to utilise the body of current knowledge, research and reliable websites that are available to support women and professionals as they consider the problems and benefits associated with breastfeeding. Methods and strategies to support the initiation and continuation of breastfeeding through the first year of an infant's life are also considered.

Although interest in the benefits of breast milk is increasing, and breastfeeding rates are correspondingly rising at a steady pace, in many countries there are unfortunately sectors in society that remain at the edge of this change, while in others a trend away from formula feeding and towards breastfeeding is still not apparent. A common goal is to increase breastfeeding rates substantially over the coming years. If there is to be any hope of moving away from the entrenched formula feeding habits of the past, healthcare professionals in all countries need to expend sustained and continuous effort to encourage women to engage fully with the infant feeding debate and with the practice of breastfeeding.

Formula milk companies are part of a global manufacturing business, the aim of which is to generate large profit margins. It is therefore a given that in the past, present and for the foreseeable future, these companies will utilise aggressive marketing strategies to promote their infant feeding products. The powerful political and economic push by the formula companies, both in the developed world and more recently in the developing world, has been a consistent force that has led to the social acceptance and normalisation of formula feeding rather than breastfeeding.

It is not surprising that professionals have found this situation difficult to compete with, and the result is a generation of women worldwide who have a predisposition towards formula feeding. The current situation poses significant challenges for professionals who support women as they consider the infant feeding options that are available, and women who are trying to make the right personal decision about infant feeding. An additional challenge for women and professionals alike is the complexity of social, cultural, political and economic factors, with potential for information overload, and being surrounded by a sea of continually changing attitudes and values.

The force of this change is reflected in the marketing practices of the major formula companies, which are turning their attention to marketing formula for older children, rather than for babies under 1 year of age. This has to be viewed as a major coup for leading organisations such as the World Health Organization (WHO) and the United Nations Children's Fund (UNICEF), formerly known as the United Nations International Children's Emergency Fund, and for the many professionals in different countries who are committed to supporting and promoting breastfeeding. Recent high-profile convictions in China linked to the adulteration of formula milk have contributed to the changing patterns of infant feeding in favour of breast milk.

A fundamental premise of this book is that healthcare professionals need to be effective information givers and to engage actively in dialogue with women at the time when those women are making key choices about infant feeding. The many issues that are central to the decisions that women make about infant feeding are addressed in different ways in the six chapters of this book.

➤ There is now a plethora of information available to women that, with only a few exceptions, provides evidence that breast milk is the best form of infant food.
➤ Professionals have access to clear, evidence-based information on the basis of which they can advise women.
➤ Breastfeeding has health benefits for both baby and mother.
➤ Formula milk has and will continue to play a useful part in infant feeding choices.
➤ Women should be in a position to make informed choices about infant feeding.
➤ Professionals should be knowledgeable and experienced in helping women to consider the controversial areas of infant feeding.
➤ Women should not be or feel pressurised to breastfeed.

Attention is also drawn to the efficiency and effectiveness of healthcare services involved in promoting and supporting the initiation and continuation of breastfeeding. Success in these endeavours is dependent on understanding what women feel and think about breastfeeding, and what they perceive it to be, and the personal and social factors that affect decisions as to whether to breastfeed. A central feature of the book is therefore the use of short vignettes taken from the qualitative research work of one of the authors, Janet Dalzell, which included interviews with women from socially deprived backgrounds, and with health professionals working in clinical maternity services and community nursing services.

The Dalzell research was completed in 2006 and has been utilised in a review and redesign of local breastfeeding services to ensure that they are more meaningful and supportive to professionals and women. The vignettes, which are scattered throughout Chapters 2, 3 and 4, reflect the real-life experiences of women using healthcare services. These chapters also conclude with examples of improvement methodology for professionals, and links to professional practice improvement tools, which can be adapted for use in different local contexts to examine and change breastfeeding policy and practice, if required.

CHAPTER SUMMARIES

Chapter 1: Exploring the politics and practices of breastfeeding

This chapter discusses the significance of a range of global policy documents that have influenced the progress made by governments and the healthcare professions in protecting, promoting and supporting breastfeeding over the last 30 years. Policy and practice are discussed in the context of international codes of practice and globally applied definitions such as exclusive breastfeeding. Included in this chapter is information on the WHO/UNICEF *Ten Steps*, the *Baby-Friendly Hospital Initiative* and the *Seven Point Plan*. The chapter concludes with a discussion of future challenges.

Chapter 2: The promotion of breastfeeding: a time and a need to change

This chapter begins with an exploration of the 'how' and 'why' of breastfeeding promotion, and establishes a link between the promotion of breastfeeding and professional assessment, with the aim of initiating and setting a firm foundation for the continuation of breastfeeding. Issues such as professional knowledge and competence, the relationship between choosing breastfeeding and self-efficacy, and the concept of 'embodied knowledge' are explored in relation to promotion of breastfeeding. Psychosocial, economic and political barriers to breastfeeding are also considered. The chapter concludes with an example of a practice improvement model.

Chapter 3: Initiating breastfeeding: a time for change – listening to the experiences of mothers

This chapter builds on the framework of the *Ten Steps*[1] and the *Seven Point Plan*[2] to explore further the claim that the central factors in breastfeeding success are promotion and effective initiation.[3] The chapter addresses issues of concern associated with relatively low rates of breastfeeding, poor levels of success in breastfeeding, lack of knowledge and skills of professionals, and poor hospital practice. The successes of the 1990s are revisited, as are strategies to initiate breastfeeding, positioning and attachment, and assessment for positioning and attachment. The chapter also includes information on taking a lactation history, 'rooming in', bed sharing, expressing breast milk, storage and handling of human milk, and the use of artificial teats or pacifiers. This chapter also concludes with an example of a practice improvement model.

Chapter 4: Supporting the continuation of breastfeeding

This chapter continues to explore the complex and dynamic interplay between the needs of the mother, the baby and the family, as well as the push and pull effects on decision making of the socio-politico-economic world both inside and outside the family. Discussions on positioning and attachment continue from the previous chapter, and poor attachment is identified as the root cause of many of the physical problems (including engorgement and mastitis) encountered by mothers during the early weeks of breastfeeding. Commonly encountered challenges to the continuation of breastfeeding are addressed, as are issues such as the importance of the woman feeling that she is supported. A range of practical issues are discussed, such as the condition of the nipples, establishing a feeding technique, peer support and exposure to role models.

Chapter 5: Breastfeeding and nutrition

Breastfeeding is discussed in the context of being the optimal infant nutrition. The first part of the chapter focuses on infant nutrition, examining different nutritional components of breast milk and the implications for the health of the infant. Some comparisons are also made with formula milk, as relevant. The chapter then moves on to consider maternal nutrition in relation to breastfeeding, and the potential effects on the health and well-being of the breastfeeding woman. This section also considers how maternal nutrition can affect the composition of breast milk, although the levels of many vitamins and minerals are sustained in breast milk even when maternal nutrition is poor. The chapter also considers the effects of other substances which can be transferred in breast milk, such as alcohol and prescribed drugs. The chapter ends with a short discussion of antigen avoidance for those children who have or are at risk of developing atopic eczema.

Chapter 6: Towards evidence-based practice

A major challenge at the present time is the phenomenon of 'information overload.' Women who are considering their choices with regard to infant feeding, and healthcare professionals who are aiming to promote and support breastfeeding, may both find themselves with a large volume of information to consider. This chapter focuses on the importance of professionals providing women with information that is current, relevant and, importantly, based on sound research evidence. The chapter uses five case studies to demonstrate the increasingly essential role that research evidence plays for the healthcare professional, and to highlight the many different issues which need to be considered when reading and appraising research. The research studies chosen for discussion are on contemporary topics related to breastfeeding, some of which have controversial components. Collectively, these studies demonstrate how research has the potential to influence attitudes to breastfeeding either negatively or positively. They also show why it is essential for healthcare professionals to have knowledge of and competence in critiquing, interpreting and transferring research results, and in using research evidence to develop professional practice and enhance the quality of healthcare services that are delivered to patients and clients.

Further reading

Each chapter ends with suggestions for further reading, all of which are available online. These have been included to support extension of learning in particular aspects of breastfeeding.

REFERENCES

1 UNICEF/World Health Organization. *The UNICEF Baby-Friendly Hospital Initiative: ten steps to successful breastfeeding.* New York: UNICEF; 1992.
2 UNICEF. *Baby-Friendly Initiative: a seven point plan for the protection, promotion and support of breastfeeding in community health settings.* London: UNICEF; 1999.
3 World Health Organization. *Protecting, Promoting and Supporting Breastfeeding: the role of maternity services.* Geneva: World Health Organization; 1989.

CHAPTER 1

Exploring the politics and practices of breastfeeding

The WHO resolutions since the early 1980s reflect the complex array of psychological, political, social and economic factors associated with the desirable changes in breastfeeding policy and practice.

Contemporary examples exist in research, policy and practice, in different countries, which demonstrate continuation of the fundamental work carried out in the last two decades of the twentieth century. [1]

INTRODUCTION

This chapter explores aspects of breastfeeding policy and practice, with particular emphasis on international codes of practice and other global policy statements that aim to influence and guide interest and action with regard to the protection, promotion and support of breastfeeding. International directives and statements are explored in the context of their impact on best practices in breastfeeding, at national and local levels.

DIFFERENT LEVELS OF POLITICAL INTEREST

International level

Political interest in breastfeeding at an international level is clearly in evidence from the 1980s onwards. Major organisations such as the World Health Organization (WHO), UNICEF and the World Health Assembly (WHA) played a key role in leading this international effort. This effort was sustained throughout the 1980s and early 1990s through a range of key meetings and the global dissemination of key policy statements and guidelines. The result was that a number of governments included the proactive promotion of breastfeeding as part of health policy.

National level

This international action was juxtaposed with a range of different national partnerships and practices designed to achieve change. The last three decades (1980–2010) have therefore demonstrated the potential benefits of collaborative professional, academic and research activities, which complemented the international effort. This collective effort with regard to breastfeeding in many countries, such as the UK and Australia, led to major new practice initiatives and the publication of seminal research work. Several robust and reliable systematic reviews have helped to consolidate the changes that have occurred over three decades.[1-3] In addition, this concerted effort, supported by leading social and health organisations, has gently coerced governments, quasi-governmental organisations and other relevant bodies to engage with and support the breastfeeding debate.[4]

National examples exist in research, policy and practice in different countries. For example, in Hong Kong research studies demonstrate success in breastfeeding for 6 months or longer. In one study. a relatively small sample of 17 mothers revealed four themes as relevant to women's experiences:[5]

1 making the decision
2 maintaining family harmony
3 overcoming barriers
4 sustaining lactation.

Local level

As with international and national strategic policy, local policy and practice are strongly influenced by social, cultural, economic and political factors. The major practice change at local level is the top-down implementation of Baby-Friendly policies and practices in hospitals and in community healthcare facilities. Local political interest can also support bottom-up change, through many individualised examples of best practice. An example of this type of local interest can be found in the historical annuals of Dundee, in Scotland. This city has a long history of heavy (jute) and light (electronics) industry and of women contributing to the labour market. Records from the Dundee City Archives show that in 1906 the city established a special 'restaurant' for nursing mothers (mothers who were breastfeeding) where they could receive a 'nourishing' meal.[6] It was concluded that the aim of this action was to keep nursing mothers working.

However, the contemporary challenge at all levels is summed up by the European Commission, which expressed concerns that despite the plethora of activity during the 1980s and 1990s, there remain significant difficulties in interpreting the available data, and that exclusivity and duration rates of breastfeeding in virtually every country worldwide, including EU countries, fall short of the recommended levels.[7] In some EU countries, initiation rates are very low, but even in countries where these rates are relatively high, there is a significant fall during the first 6 months of breastfeeding, and the exclusive breastfeeding rate at 6 months is low throughout most of Europe.[8] The last two decades therefore appear to show a mixed picture of policy into action, and although awareness and commitment to breastfeeding are in evidence, the full impact of policy into practice has yet to be seen.

A major global challenge of the twenty-first century is that despite the mounting evidence that 'breast is best', breastfeeding is not the preferred choice of women, and breastfeeding rates remain relatively low worldwide, and are slow to rise. The reasons for this state of affairs are complex, they differ from one country to another, and they are strongly influenced by specific national and local factors. In the developed world, changing the attitudes of women is a necessity and remains a challenge, while in the developing world cause and effect can often be laid at the door of very basic issues, such as infection and illness in the mother, availability of clean water or, in some countries, scarcity of water.

INTERNATIONAL ACTIVITY: POLICY INTO PRACTICE, THE EARLY YEARS

The 33rd World Health Assembly

In October 1979 a four-day joint WHA and UNICEF meeting was held on 'Infant and Young Child Feeding.' This was attended by representatives of governments, the United Nations (UN), system and technical agencies, non-government organisations (NGOs) and the infant food industry, as well as by scientists working in this field. The main achievements and benefits of the 1979 meeting were threefold, namely to bring together a diverse mix of groups with a vested interest in breastfeeding, to ensure that breastfeeding was moved to the top of the global political agenda, and to raise awareness of the need for concerted action.

The 1979 WHA/UNICEF meeting agreed three key actions. First, it was agreed that there was an urgent need to review the existing legislation in different countries, with the specific purpose of better enabling and supporting women to breastfeed, especially working mothers. Secondly, it was recognised that strategies are required to strengthen the WHA's capacity to cooperate at the request of Member States in developing appropriate legislation. Thirdly, regular reporting to the WHA was agreed on the steps taken by the WHO to promote breastfeeding and to improve infant and young child feeding, as well as to evaluate the effects of all measures taken by the WHO and its Member States. This was to start from 1981 and to continue in even years thereafter.

An international marketing code (World Health Organization, 1981)

Two further major outcomes of the 1979 meeting were an agreement to develop an international code of conduct to guide countries on how infant formula should be promoted, supported and marketed, and a commitment from all countries to actively encourage and support breastfeeding. The following points represent the principal issues that all governments and other organisations attending the meeting agreed to for their respective countries:

➤ to address how breastfeeding can be encouraged and supported
➤ to promote and support appropriate weaning practices
➤ to strengthen education, training opportunities and methods of delivering appropriate information
➤ to promote the health and social status of women, so that women in turn are empowered in areas that relate to infant and young child feeding
➤ to implement appropriate marketing and distribution of breast milk substitutes
➤ to have in place a coherent food and nutrition policy that addresses the need for pregnant and lactating women to be adequately nourished.

The speed and direction of change moved the global community to produce the International Code of Marketing of Breast-Milk Substitutes, which contained a wide range of standards on the marketing of infant formula, and which aimed to curtail and address non-compliance. The Code was informed by previous international WHA resolutions, and was influenced by global concerns about the increase in infant mortality rates caused by the use of infant formula, especially in the developing world. The Code contained 10 provisions to guide the marketing of breast milk substitutes, as shown in Box 1.1.[9]

Box 1.1 Ten provisions of the International Code of Marketing of Breast-Milk Substitutes

1 No advertising of any of these products to the public.
2 No free samples to mothers.
3 No promotion of products in healthcare facilities, including no free supplies.
4 No company mothercraft nurses to advise mothers.
5 No gifts or personal samples to be given to health workers.
6 No words or pictures idealising artificial feeding, including pictures of infants, to be displayed on the labels of the products.
7 All information on artificial feeding, including the labels, should explain the benefits of breastfeeding, and the costs and hazards associated with artificial feeding.
8 Unsuitable products such as sweetened condensed milk should not be promoted for babies.
9 All products should be of a high quality.
10 Quality should take account of the climatic storage conditions of the country in which the products are used.

The 1981 Code aimed to control practices related to the international marketing of breast milk substitutes and thereby to protect all mothers and babies from inappropriate company practices in promoting breast milk substitutes.[10] It aimed to ensure that women receive accurate information about breastfeeding, but equally important, it aimed to ban the promotion of baby milks and other breast milk substitutes.

The Code was adopted and supported by law in many countries. Taylor found that in some countries the 1981 Code was given legal backing to increase compliance.[11] For example, in the 1980s the Hong Kong government prohibited advertisements of infant formula through the mass media.

Clear evidence of developments since the 1979 WHA/UNICEF meeting can be found in numerous policy statements from the early 1980s to the present day, from global organisations such as WHO and UNICEF. These statements demonstrate a clear commitment among powerful and influential organisations to the promotion, protection and support of breastfeeding. The key issues are covered in a number of WHA resolutions issued during the 1980s. These address infant nutrition and appropriate feeding practices for infants and young children, and include resolutions WHA33.32, WHA34.22, WHA35.26, WHA37.30, WHA39.28, WHA41.11, WHA43.3, WHA45.34, WHA46.7, WHA47.5 and WHA49.15. The WHA resolutions can be found at www.breastfeedingalberta.ca/resolutions.htm

The impact of the WHA resolutions

Responsibility for implementing the recommendations of the various WHA resolutions was recognised as needing to be shared between health services, health personnel, national governments and authorities, women's and other non-government organisations, the agencies of the UN and the infant food industry. These resolutions recognised that decisions about infant feeding made by a woman and her family raise a number of physical, social and emotional challenges. The global and national issues addressed in WHA resolutions during the 1980s and 1990s can be summarised as follows:

➤ the need for close consultation of all interested groups
➤ prompt action when required and on specifically targeted areas
➤ safe and adequate nutrition for infants and young children
➤ provision of adequate and relevant information
➤ active promotion of breastfeeding
➤ proper use of breast-milk substitutes
➤ attention to the education and training needs of healthcare professionals
➤ attention to policy and practice in relation to the adequate production, storage and distribution of breast-milk substitutes
➤ development of international quality standards
➤ promotion of the harmonious physical and psychosocial development of the child
➤ support for and encouragement of the use of local products in weaning
➤ a major review of advertising codes and legislation relating to the sales of baby foods
➤ adequate support for mothers who are working away from their homes during the lactation period

➤ intensification of activities in the field of health education, training and information about infant and young child feeding.

INTERNATIONAL ACTIVITY: POLICY INTO PRACTICE IN THE 1990s

Towards the end of the 1980s, policy guidelines moved closer to strategy implementation of best practice in breastfeeding at a local level, in the form of the Ten Steps identified as necessary to successful breastfeeding (*see* Box 1.2).[12] The Ten Steps confirmed the commitment of leading global health organisations to protecting, promoting and supporting breastfeeding, and aimed to guide maternity services in developing policy and practice in the key areas that support breastfeeding.

Box 1.2 Ten Steps to Successful Breastfeeding

1 Have a written breastfeeding policy that is routinely communicated to all healthcare staff.
2 Train all healthcare staff in the skills necessary to implement the breastfeeding policy.
3 Inform all pregnant women about the benefits and management of breastfeeding.
4 Help mothers to initiate breastfeeding soon after birth.
5 Show mothers how to breastfeed and how to maintain lactation even if they are separated from their babies.
6 Give newborn infants no food or drink other than breast milk, unless medically indicated.
7 Practise rooming in, allowing mothers and infants to remain together 24 hours a day.
8 Encourage breastfeeding on demand.
9 Give no artificial teats or dummies to breastfeeding infants.
10 Foster the establishment of breastfeeding support groups, and refer mothers to them on discharge from the hospital or clinic.

The Innocenti Declaration (1990)

The Ten Steps acted as a trigger to actions in other countries that were designed to protect, promote and support breastfeeding. The Innocenti Declaration was produced and adopted by participants at the Spedale degli Innocenti in Italy, in 1990. (The Spedale degli Innocenti or 'Hospital of the Innocents' is a children's orphanage in Florence that is dedicated to supporting and protecting poor children.)

The Innocenti document upholds the uniqueness of the breastfeeding process, and outlines the required changes and operational targets that governments should aim to achieve in order to protect, promote and support breastfeeding. It has been influential in reinforcing the need for professional and government involvement in the promotion of breastfeeding, in creating opportunities to breastfeed and in assisting women to breastfeed successfully. The operational recommendations of the Innocenti Declaration are listed in Box 1.3.

Box 1.3 Recommendations of the Innocenti Declaration

- Appoint a national breastfeeding coordinator and establish a multisectoral national breastfeeding committee.
- Ensure that all facilities that provide maternity services fully practise all of the Ten Steps to Successful Breastfeeding as set out by the WHO/UNICEF document *Protecting, Promoting and Supporting Breastfeeding: the special role of the maternity services.*
- Take action to give effect to the principles and aims of all Articles of the International Code of Marketing of Breast-Milk Substitutes (1981).
- Enable imaginative legislation to protect the breastfeeding rights of working women and establish means for its enforcement.
- Support national situation analysis and surveys and the development of national goals and targets for action.
- Encourage and support national authorities in planning, implementing, monitoring and evaluating their breastfeeding policies.

The Innocenti Declaration constituted an important international policy statement on breastfeeding. It aimed to change attitudes towards breastfeeding practice worldwide, and was adopted by participating governments and WHO/UNICEF policy makers. It is considered to be a pivotal force in influencing breastfeeding on a global scale.

The Baby-Friendly Hospital Initiative (1991)

The baby-friendly concept evolved into a second strategy, which was supported globally, that aimed to further reinforce the best practices in breastfeeding initiated in the Ten Steps. The idea of hospitals that were managed and operated according to baby-friendly standards and criteria was launched at the International Paediatric Association Conference in Ankara in 1991, and was established in 1992, to take forward the Innocenti Declaration and the Ten Steps.[13]

The Seven Point Plan

The success of the Baby-Friendly Initiative in hospitals was demonstrated by its extension from hospital to community practice. Fundamental to the Baby-Friendly Initiative in the community is the *Seven Point Plan for Sustaining Breastfeeding in the Community*. The Seven Point Plan was the outcome of a widespread consultation with healthcare professionals, service providers and users, and it reflects the consensus as to what constitutes best practice in community health services. It is outlined in Box 1.4.

Box 1.4 The Seven Point Plan

1 Have in place a written breastfeeding policy that is routinely communicated to all healthcare staff.
2 Train all staff involved in the care of mothers and babies in the skills necessary to implement the policy.
3 Inform all antenatal women about the benefits and management of breastfeeding.
4 Support mothers to initiate and sustain breastfeeding.
5 Encourage exclusive and continued breastfeeding, with appropriately timed introduction of complementary foods.
6 Provide a welcoming atmosphere for breastfeeding families.
7 Promote cooperation between healthcare staff, breastfeeding support groups and the local community.

The Seven Points were subsequently revised in 2008.[14] The revision document can be accessed at www.babyfriendly.org.uk/pdfs/The_Seven_Point_Plan_September_2008.pdf

Healthcare professionals in the UK expected, required and received government support for the changes in policy and practice relating to the initiation of baby-friendly practices.[15] The widespread adoption of the Baby-Friendly Initiative, the Ten Steps and the Seven Point Plan in the UK and other countries is an excellent example of what can be achieved through cooperation at international, national and local levels where professionals, supported by global health organisations and their governments, take the lead in key policy areas that require change.

Examples of Baby-Friendly Initiative and Seven Point Plan developments can be found at the following Canadian and Australian websites:

➤ Breastfeeding Committee for Canada: www.breastfeedingcanada.ca/html/webdoc43.html
➤ Australian College of Midwives: http://acmi.naqtechnology.com.au/Portals/8/position%20statements/DRAFT%20Position%20Statement%20on%20Infant%20Feeding.pdf.

The Seven Point Plan and the Ten Steps complement each other. They represent a giant step forward in terms of supporting and sustaining breastfeeding. Their implementation goes a long way towards ensuring that women are well informed about infant feeding choices, and that professional practice in hospital and community healthcare meets a quality standard of care for all women. Together they provide a framework that supports best practice, guides the development of care standards and, importantly, facilitates the continuous development of policy and practice.

A professional account of a journey to establish the Baby-Friendly Initiative in Ontario, Canada, can be found at www.beststart.org/events/detail/bsannual-conf07/presentations/preconf/P1_5.pdf

INTERNATIONAL ACTIVITY: POLICY INTO PRACTICE FROM 2000

The developments of the 1980s and 1990s continually sustained and reinforced the international consensus that breastfeeding was the best option for infants, especially for the first 6 months of life. By the early 2000s, more than 15 000 hospitals around the world had been officially designated as baby-friendly, and many countries have developed national action plans and policies to support the global recognition and value of breastfeeding.[16]

North America

Practice was supported in the USA through the breastfeeding policy 'Blueprint for Action.'[17] This included an action plan related to supporting breastfeeding based on education, training, awareness, support and research. The Blueprint document contains key recommendations for improvements in baby-friendly practices in the hospital setting, in the workplace, in the support of families and communities and in research. These elements form a formidable and strong formula that supports breastfeeding.

The USA also replaced a previous statement published in 1997 with a new policy statement in February 2005 by the American Academy of Pediatrics (AAP) on 'Breastfeeding and the Use of Human Milk.'[18] The 2005 document contains a wide range of reference sources, which reflect the growing body of knowledge on the benefits of breastfeeding and clinical management. It also includes issues relevant to high-risk infants, recommendations on the role of the healthcare professional, and a statement on research.

Europe

In Europe a similar approach to the Blueprint in the USA was adopted, with representation from the European Union (EU) members. This EU project for the promotion of breastfeeding in Europe published the document *Protection, Promotion and Support of Breastfeeding in Europe: a blueprint for action.*[19] This provides a model for regional and national planning, with recommendations for action.

The 54th World Health Assembly (2001)

Two important agenda areas for the new century brought forward by the 54th WHA were exclusive breastfeeding and the International Code of Marketing of Breast-Milk Substitutes. At the 2001 Assembly there was global consensus on the need for exclusive breastfeeding, and because this is considered by the WHO to be a crucial public health issue, it is kept continually under review.[20] The Assembly considered the optimal duration of exclusive breastfeeding under the Global Strategy for Infant and Young Child Feeding. This Assembly also marked the 20th anniversary of the adoption of the International Code of Marketing of Breast-Milk Substitutes. Resolution 54.2 considered past WHA resolutions on infant nutrition and appropriate feeding practices for infants and young children, and reinforced resolutions on the International Code's fundamental role of protecting, promoting and supporting breastfeeding. This meeting also gave due consideration to the need for international and national commitment to support for working women to breastfeed.

The practical value of research

The 2001 Assembly also debated the availability of scientific research on the balance of risk of HIV transmission through breastfeeding. The need for further research associated with the nutrition of infants of HIV-positive mothers was recognised. Based on existing evidence, it was agreed that when replacement feeding is safe, affordable and sustainable, HIV-positive women should be advised not to breastfeed. In addition, exclusive breastfeeding is recommended during the first months of life, and decisions to use formula feeding should be free from commercial influences. More information about the WHO recommendations on HIV and breastfeeding can be found online at http://whqlibdoc.who.int/hq/2003/9241591226.pdf.

Concerns were also raised at the Assembly that policy decisions (and, by implication, practice) continue to be hampered by lack of conclusive, global research evidence.[21] Although the criticisms relating to research are timely and fair, it is also important to recognise that research in the areas related to baby-friendliness has achieved a great deal in bridging the divide between research and practice.

Two major recommendations were proposed to guide consistency between policy, practice and research. First, exclusive breastfeeding should continue for 6 months, with the introduction of complementary foods following this 6-month period, alongside continued breastfeeding. Secondly, more attention to the nutritional status of pregnant and lactating mothers and to the prevalence of deficiencies of micronutrients such as iron, zinc, and vitamin A was needed.

Consensus was reached that the main purpose of research should be to inform practice. The priority research areas recommended by the Assembly included a comparison of exclusive breastfeeding/predominant breastfeeding and partial breastfeeding for 4 to 6 months based on the following outcomes:[22]

➤ proportion of infants with growth faltering and malnutrition at 6 and 12 months
➤ micronutrient status
➤ diarrhoeal morbidity
➤ neuromotor development
➤ changes in weight in mothers
➤ lactational amenorrhoea in mothers
➤ clarification of the range (globally) of biological and social factors that mitigate against exclusive breastfeeding to 6 months, in order to identify barriers and design appropriate and effective interventions.

Infant and young child feeding

The momentum of change was given a further boost in the early 2000s with the publication of the *WHO Global Strategy for Infant and Young Child Feeding*. This strategy document aimed to raise awareness around the world of the way in which feeding choices and practices for babies and young children affect their health and well-being. Furthermore, as a global public health recommendation, the WHO declared for the first time that during the first 6 months of life babies should be exclusively breastfed in order to attain the best possible health, growth and development.[23]

The 61st World Health Assembly (2008)

The work of the WHA to protect and support women with regard to breastfeeding continues through a range of documents and resolutions aimed at guiding policy and practice. At the 61st WHA, resolution 61.15, agenda item 11.7, in considering the Global Immunisation Strategy, made reference to the importance of breast-feeding for the development of the baby's immune system. This new resolution WHA 61.15 urged Member States to '. . . strengthen efforts to protect, promote and support early and effective breastfeeding, in order to boost the development of infants' overall immune system (p. 2).[24]

WHERE WILL THE FUTURE CHALLENGES COME FROM?

Various key documents, codes and guidelines from the WHA, the WHO and other leading international organisations and groups provide a strong foundation for policy and practice in the future, in both the developed and the developing worlds. Sustained effort by governments and industry, as well as by the professions, to gain a global level of commitment to exclusive breastfeeding for the first 6 months of an infant's life and restrict the marketing of formula is now well established policy and practice in many countries.

Unfortunately, the codes and guidelines are not applied uniformly throughout the world, and in many countries they are still simply ignored. At the end of the 1990s the *British Medical Journal (BMJ)* reported that in nearly all of the 31 countries surveyed there was non-compliance with the WHO code from the main producers of infant formula and other breast-milk substitutes.[25] This conclusion was supported by research evidence from the Interagency Group on Breastfeeding Monitoring of UNICEF, which also found violations of the code in Bangladesh, Poland, South Africa and Thailand.[26.]

In addition, the leading organisations and agencies spearheading this movement do not have legal power to enforce the codes or guidelines. On the one hand, progress seems to be dependent on the degree of beneficence within governments to support this important healthcare change, while on the other hand, progress is held to ransom by governments that are uncaring or, worse still, malevolent towards women and infants. Undoubtedly, future challenges will be inextricably linked with political, economic and ethical considerations.

In countries where the threat of adulteration is negligible, other unethical marketing practices have been observed. These include inducements to health professionals to recommend formula feeding bottles, and free trial supplies of milk substitutes to mothers.

As recent events have testified, the threat of catastrophic consequences caused by adulteration during the manufacturing and production processes of formula milk remains very real. In April 2004 the Chinese authorities arrested 22 manufacturers of baby milk and closed three factories because they had sold fake products, which had caused more than 12 infant deaths and hundreds of cases of malnourishment. Some of the products had only 6% of the required nutritional value, and some were found to contain no more nutrient value than water. Many infants suffered from a range of conditions associated with under-nourishment and severe malnutrition, which resulted not only in suffering but also in chronic, long-term conditions.[27] China is not the only culprit. In late 2004 the German company Humana Milchunion also paid out approximately $20 000 000 to Israeli families whose children had suffered major neurological damage due to feeding with thiamine-deficient formula.[28]

In September 2008, history repeated itself. Infant milk formula produced in China and distributed within China, Bangladesh, Burundi, Myanmar, Gabon and Yemen was found to contain lethal doses of melamine, an industrial chemical used in plastic. In September 2008 the Ministry of Health of China confirmed that the adulteration had caused the death of three babies, and over 6240 infants were found to have kidney stones, a very rare condition in infants. Apparently the General Administration of Quality Supervision, Inspection and Quarantine (GAQSIQ) in China, which is responsible for checking milk and related merchandise, had been aware of the illegal use of melamine for a long time and was unable to prevent this recent catastrophe.[29] At least 22 dairy manufacturers across the country were found to have melamine in some of their products, with levels ranging from 0.09 mg/kg to 2.56 mg/kg.[30]

Siegel-Itzkovich, commenting on the adulteration of formula in 2004, stated that although the problem remained a contemporary one, the evidence suggests that governments and the legal profession are waking up to the scale of the problem and its relevance to the health of infants.[31] Sadly, this is not the case. The 2008 episode in China demonstrates that ruthless individuals are willing, and more importantly able, to break both the letter and the spirit of the WHO 1981 code. Rather than waking up to the scale of the problem, as Siegel-Itzkovich suggests, some governments appear to be sleeping on the job of monitoring production to the rigorous standards set out in the Code. Governments therefore need to be more aware that unscrupulous producers of formula milk are undeterred and are willing to risk severe penalties, endangering the lives of vulnerable infants, for the sake of high profit margins. Governments and the healthcare professions thus have good cause to remain concerned and vigilant about the ability of the Code to regulate the quality of formula milk production and distribution worldwide.

For those manufacturers of infant formula who scrupulously observe product quality standards, profit margins continue to drive aggressive marketing techniques and the over-promotion of products. Ironically, in the developing world mothers and mothers-to-be, who are already poor, are encouraged to pay for food for their baby or babies, when it could be supplied by their own body, without cost. According to Dykes, the cost of formula can often use up to 30% of a family's income in the developing world, and can have an impact on the calorie intake of the rest of the family.[32] Mothers who abandon breastfeeding become the captive market of the formula companies, and the effects go beyond the mother and her family. The costs associated with introducing formula feeding are not just those of the formula milk itself, but also include items such as bottles,

TABLE 1.1 Percentage of infants breastfed immediately postpartum compared with the percentage exclusively breastfed at 6 months

Country	Early postpartum (%)	Exclusively at 6 months (%)
USA	74	12
UK	76	3
Canada	87	16

TABLE 1.2 Percentage of infants breastfed exclusively at 6 months

Country	Exclusively at 6 months (%)
China	51
Chile	63
Cuba	41
Egypt	38
India	46
Kenya	13
Malawi	56
Mexico	38
Nigeria	17
South Africa	7
Thailand	5
Turkey	21
Zimbabwe	22

teats and sterilising equipment, as well as increased healthcare costs associated with additional hospitalisation, problems of dehydration and contraception.[33]

For various reasons the percentage of infants who are breastfeeding exclusively remains a cause for concern, and is an area that needs to be addressed in the future. Tables 1.1 and 1.2 demonstrate the variations from one country to another with regard to exclusive breastfeeding at 6 months. The interpretation of data and comparative data analysis are hampered by the lack of availability of reliable data and the lack of systematic methods for collecting data. Tables 1.1 and 1.2 are based on information from the following sources:

➤ UNICEF: www.unicef.org/infobycountry/index.html
➤ UK Infant Feeding Survey 2005: www.ic.nhs.uk/statistics-and-data-collections/health-and-lifestyles-related-surveys/infant-feeding-survey/infant-feeding-survey-2005
➤ US Centers for Disease Control and Prevention (CDC): www.cdc.gov/breastfeeding/data/NIS_data/
➤ Canadian Perinatal Health Report 2008: www.phac-aspc.gc.ca/publicat/2008/cphr-rspc/index-eng.php.

It is suggested that the healthcare budgets in developed countries could be substantially reduced if approximately three-quarters of women in a country breastfeed, and the majority of this number breastfeed for 6 months. It has been estimated that a minimum of $3.6 billion would be saved if breastfeeding was to be increased from current levels (64% in hospital, and 29% at 6 months) to those recommended by the US Surgeon General (75% and 50%, respectively). This figure is likely to be an underestimate of the total savings, because it represents cost savings from the treatment of only three childhood illnesses (otitis media, gastroenteritis and necrotising enterocolitis).[34]

CONCLUSION

It is clear that protecting, promoting and supporting mothers with regard to initiation and continuation of breastfeeding remains an international policy priority, which is strongly linked to the continuous development of national and local practices in breastfeeding, and the growth of research related to breastfeeding. Over a generation, considerable and concerted effort has gone into producing and implementing policies and practices associated with the Baby-Friendly Initiative and other landmark initiatives such as the Ten Steps and the Seven Point Plan. This effort has provided a firm foundation for future action in the twenty-first century.

This first chapter identifies that the extent to which women and families are informed and supported with regard to breastfeeding, and how well breastfeeding interests are promoted and protected and 'best practice' is facilitated, are dependent on the interpretation and implementation of policy and practice at the local level. Effective local policy and practice therefore reflect the ethical and professional values, principles and standards that operate in a specific region or healthcare facility. In addition, professionals with a role in supporting and promoting breastfeeding cannot escape the accompanying political challenges and the degree to which political awareness is beneficial for influencing and implementing change.

Inevitably, women are at the centre of breastfeeding activity and should be protected and supported in making informed choices about the type of infant feeding that they wish to adopt. This creates different challenges for healthcare professionals and governments across the globe, starting from the basic principle that women and young children have a fundamental human right to protection and benevolent policy making by governments, including protection and support for breastfeeding. The above conclusions are illustrated in Figure 1.1.

For professionals, the challenges are undeniably many and complex, and are often linked to expertise in listening, information management and information giving. For example, it has been reported that some professionals may be fearful about asking women outright to state their intentions with regard to infant feeding, because of concerns that once a woman has stated her intention to use formula, the door to further information and discussion about breastfeeding will be partially or completely closed.[35] However, there is a growing body of guidelines, research evidence and systematic reviews on breastfeeding, which can be used by healthcare professionals to inform and support women who are making decisions about infant feeding. Fortunately, the professional effort today to support, protect and promote breastfeeding continues with the same high level of intensity that has been demonstrated since the early 1980s.

The website of the National Conference of State Legislatures in the USA (www.ncsl.org/programs/health/breast50.htm) provides information about the

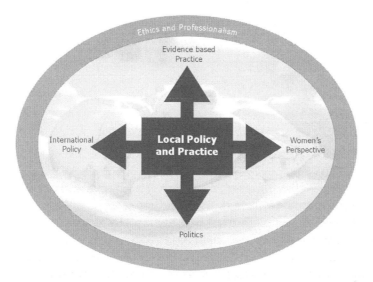

FIGURE 1.1: Local policy and practice.

legal issues to which various US states have committed, in relation to supporting breastfeeding. In 2009, the National Conference of State Legislatures also stated its aim of increasing the percentage of women who breastfeed during the postpartum period to 75% by 2010.[36]

In this age of readily available information from online sources, popular sites such as YouTube demonstrate en masse the force of public opinion for breastfeeding. In 2009, a YouTube video (which can be viewed at www.birthactivist. com/2009/03/hong-kong-government-tackles-public-breastfeeding) drew public attention to the issue of breastfeeding in public in Hong Kong, and the lack of provision of adequate facilities for mothers to breastfeed outside the home.

EXAMPLE OF A POLITICAL CHALLENGE

A large number of community staff were interested in and committed to the implementation of the UNICEF Community Baby-Friendly Initiative. A formal approach to gain approval by the organisation can be a useful and productive approach to influence and negotiate change.

Using a strategy paper to address the challenge

The paper provided as an example can be used as a template to initiate change at the highest levels when recommending particular strategies or initiatives, which will benefit service users, in this case pregnant women and new mothers. There may also be a need to overcome opinion-based decisions by providing clear evidence for change.

The first reference point for those involved in this change activity was the *Ten Steps to Successful Breastfeeding*, to provide a framework for further discussion about building evidence to support their recommendations. It would also be used in the implementation of evidence-based practice, which is sensitive to the needs of women and is recommended in both national and local policy documents.

The example paper can be used to provide insight for senior managers, leaders and stakeholders. Such papers can be used to explore and highlight the ethical and political issues that are relevant to those who manage and fund services.

A strategy paper for implementing the WHO/UNICEF Community Baby-Friendly Initiative in xxx

1 **Purpose of the report**
   The xxx Committee are asked to support in principle and provide key professional leadership for this initiative in their health/medical centres. Details of the process and implication are included in this report.

2 **Recommendations**
   The xxx Committee approves the future development of the Hospital Baby-Friendly Initiative/Community Baby-Friendly Initiative with xxx Hospital *or* a cluster of interested general practices in each xxx area/community.

3 Executive summary

Breastfeeding is a public health priority throughout xxx. The WHO/UNICEF Baby-Friendly Hospital Initiative has successfully been implemented in xxx and is currently being progressed in xxx Hospital. Babies born in Baby-Friendly Accredited Hospitals in xxx are 28% more likely to be exclusively breastfeeding at 7 days and have significant improvements in breastfeeding rates over time. The Community Baby-Friendly Initiative has the potential to support the duration of breastfeeding for this increasing number of mothers choosing to breastfeed in xxx. The Community Baby-Friendly Initiative involves the implementation of evidence-based practice standards for the care of pregnant and postnatal women, as supported in the breastfeeding policy for xxx. The implementation of the practice standards leads to a prestigious nationally recognised quality award in recognition of the significant contribution to supporting breastfeeding in general practice populations.

The xxx clinical standards for maternity services published in xxx ask healthcare providers to provide evidence that the maternity service adheres to the principles of, or is working towards, the UNICEF/WHO Baby-Friendly status, which includes primary care services. Xxx will be assessed in xxx for evidence of these standards being progressed in all areas of xxx.

4 Financial implications

There is a small programme budget allocation to develop resources required for implementation. Training will be provided by members of the xxx Strategy Group, and negotiation will take place to release staff via the practice-based protected learning time or by appropriately trained practice staff (e.g. health visitors). It is anticipated that the cost of an external assessment by UNICEF would be met by xxx.

5 Risk assessment

The health benefits for mothers and infants are globally recognised. All continued progress would contribute towards the national health targets for breastfeeding. A full risk assessment has been performed and coded as red, which indicates that it is unlikely that improvement in breastfeeding initiation and continuation rates will take place unless there is a concentrated focus involving both hospital and community.

6 Implications for health

The national target is for more than xxx% of mothers still to be breastfeeding their baby at 6 weeks of age by xxx. Data provided from various sources indicate that continuation levels at 6–8 weeks have increased very slightly in xxx from x% to x% since xxx. It therefore seems highly unlikely that, if current trends continue, the national and local targets will be met by xxx, and further action must be taken.

There is significant and reliable evidence that breastfeeding has important advantages for both the infant and the mother. The xxx Infant Feeding Study indicated in 1990 that breastfeeding rates were highest in social groups I to III, with no exclusive breastfeeding taking place in social class V. Almost

20 years later the xxx Strategy for xxx identified that this trend continued into the early 2000s, with breastfeeding rates on discharge from hospital ranging from x% in the most disadvantaged areas to x% in the more affluent areas of xxx. There is clear evidence that the health of children is improved regardless of social class groups if they have been breastfed, with recommendations to target breastfeeding interventions in low-income groups as part of the xxx Strategy. Protective benefits for the infant include reduced risk of gastrointestinal infection, respiratory infections, necrotising enterocolitis, urinary tract infections, otitis media, allergic disease (eczema, asthma and wheezing) and insulin-dependent diabetes mellitus. Women who breastfeed are at lower risk of breast cancer, ovarian cancer and hip fractures. Increasing rates will improve long-term health for mothers and their infants. Where the Community Baby-Friendly Initiative is implemented there is a reduced rate of consultation with GPs about common childhood illnesses.

7 **Timetable for implementation and Lead Officer**

Approval will enable xxx Hospital *or* interested GP practices/medical centres to participate in the implementation of the Community Baby-Friendly Initiative. The xxx Directorate will support a baseline audit of current practice, and this will inform the development of an action plan, including a timetable for commencing in spring xxx. Further information about the process is included in Section 9.

8 **Consultation**

In xxx a paper was presented and considered by the conference members who supported the recommendations for implementation of the Community Baby-Friendly Initiative in principle. Discussions then took place with the general managers of the xxx areas, who asked for detailed information about the work required for this initiative in order for the xxx committee to approve this proposal.

Discussions have also taken place with a range of healthcare professionals throughout xxx. The initiative is supported in principle by the community nurses, managers and health visitors in xxx.

9 **Background**

Despite considerable commitment to working towards the promotion, protection and support of breastfeeding locally, breastfeeding rates at 6–8 weeks have remained static since xxx in xxx. In xxx a strategy group collectively decided to review the strategic focus of breastfeeding interventions. As a result, there will be a concentrated focus on the services offered to women during pregnancy and the first 6 weeks of the postnatal period. Interventions that support this include the Baby-Friendly Hospital Initiative, the Community Baby-Friendly Initiative, a new breastfeeding training programme for midwives, health visitors and public health nurses, and various research projects.

The UK Baby-Friendly Hospital Initiative was launched in 1994. This was based on the *WHO/UNICEF Joint Declaration on the Promotion, Protection and Support of Breastfeeding: the role of the maternity services*. This led to the subsequent publication of the *Ten Steps to Successful Breastfeeding* in the hospital setting. Four years later, in 1998, the *Seven Point Plan for the Protection, Promotion and Support of Breastfeeding in Community Health Care Settings* was published by WHO/UNICEF. This complements and overlaps with the *Ten Steps* to provide agreed practice standards for pregnant and breastfeeding women, known as the Community Baby-Friendly Initiative.

The Community Baby-Friendly Initiative involves the adoption of breastfeeding policy, appropriate training of staff, supporting information giving to women during pregnancy and the initiation and duration of breastfeeding, providing a welcoming atmosphere to breastfeeding women on GP premises, and appropriate handover of care between health professionals. This involves community midwives, health visitors and general practitioners working in collaboration to achieve these practice standards. Compliance with the International Code of Marketing of Breast-Milk Substitutes is required, including withdrawal of the sale of infant formula in healthcare premises and the advertising of infant formula. Implementation of the Community Baby-Friendly Initiative would complement the strategic objectives in xxx. These standards lead to a nationally recognised quality award in recognition of the significant contribution to supporting breastfeeding in GP practice populations.

10 **What will be required by participating practices/medical centres?**
The vast majority of this initiative's work involves predominantly midwives, community midwives, health visitors and public health nurses. The greatest challenge will be the release of staff to receive necessary training appropriate to their role. This will be negotiated as part of the practice-based protected learning time for the cluster group.

- An integrated xxx policy has been ratified and approved and would need to be adopted by the participating general practices.
- With regard to training, it is anticipated that with the exception of midwives, health visitors and public health nurses, this will be provided with approval in the practice-based protected learning time. Time frames are indicated below. Relevant resources for management of breastfeeding complications would be supplied in each consulting room. Records of training will be held in each practice and by facilitators.
- Midwives, health visitors and public health nurses are required to assist women in making an informed infant feeding choice that is appropriate to their circumstances, and to ensure that they are fully supported in this decision. GPs would be required to support this process, ensuring that the information given is consistent.
- Support of women is predominantly the responsibility of midwives, health visitors and public health nurses. Where complications of breastfeeding occur, the GP is required to manage or refer the case as appropriate. Practice nurses and reception/administration staff are required to be knowledgeable about the policy, and may be required

Objective	Lead officer	Staff group	Implementation	Completion
Training	<Insert>	Practice managers	2 hours	<Insert>
		General practitioners	1 hour	
			1 hour	
		Practice nurse	1 hour	
		Reception/ administration		
Breastfeeding education	<Insert>	Midwives	18 hours	<Insert>
		Health visitors		
		Public health nurses		

to refer women to appropriate support. A postnatal checklist will be developed to assist community midwives and health visitors with regard to sharing of information.

- Encouragement of exclusive and continued breastfeeding, with appropriately timed introduction of complementary foods, is predominantly the responsibility of midwives and health visitors, but may occasionally involve GPs.
- A welcoming atmosphere should be created (display of policy, posters and information in the facility, reception/administration staff knowledgeable about policy and support of breastfeeding women) on the premises.
- With regard to breastfeeding groups, GPs, midwives, health visitors and reception/administration staff should know where to refer breastfeeding women.

<Insert similar information about local requirements for hospital criteria.>

FURTHER READING
The Ten Steps
Read about the Ten Steps and some global success stories about their implementation (www.unicef.org/programme/breastfeeding/baby.htm).

The Baby-Friendly website provides information on each of the Ten Steps, and outlines clearly for each one the associated standard, how the standard is assessed in practice, and how the standard can be assessed for compliance (www.baby friendly.org.uk/page.asp?page=60).

The Innocenti Declaration
This substantial document was published in celebration of 15 years of the Innocenti Declaration on promoting, protecting and supporting breastfeeding (www.unicef.org/nutrition/files/Innocenti_plus15_BreastfeedingReport.pdf).

The International Code of Marketing of Breast-Milk Substitutes
This website provide a useful synopsis of the WHO code (www.babymilkaction. org/regs/thecode.html).

UNICEF also provides information about the Code. (www.unicef.org/programme/ breastfeeding/code.htm).

The International Baby Food Action Network (IBFAN) is a further source of information on the code, including information on the systematic undermining of breastfeeding (www.ibfan.org/issue-international_code.html).

The Baby-Friendly Initiative
UNICEF has published a guide to implementing the Baby-Friendly best practice standards for breastfeeding in maternity and community healthcare facilities.

An implementation guide for both the Ten Steps and the Seven Point Plan has been prepared by the UNICEF UK Baby-Friendly Initiative (www.babyfriendly. org.uk). This site contains best practice standards for the support of breastfeeding (evidence, resources, training, statistics, guidance, leaflets for parents and strategies).

World Health Organization information on breastfeeding
In 2003, the WHO published their *Global Strategy for Infant and Young Child Feeding*. A summary and link to the full document are available (at www.who.int/ entity/child_adolescent_health/topics/prevention_care/child/nutrition/global).

This is a large document (157 pages) that is useful for teams of key policy makers, non-government organisations and managers of healthcare services. The document incorporates a tool (which can be found at www.who.int/child_ adolescent_health/documents/9241562544/en/index.html) that is designed to assess the strengths and weaknesses of policies and programmes for protecting, promoting and supporting optimal feeding practices in their local setting, and to determine where improvements may be needed to meet the aims and objectives of the *Global Strategy for Infant and Young Child Feeding*.

Centers for Disease Control and Prevention

The US Centers for Disease Control and Prevention (CDC) website has an area devoted to breastfeeding, which incorporates a range of useful resources and publications (www.cdc.gov/breastfeeding).

News items

The recall of contaminated formula milk in China was a major international news story in 2008. Some analyses of this news story can be found on the following websites:

➤ www.timesonline.co.uk/tol/news/world/asia/article4790866.ece
➤ www.cnn.com/2008/WORLD/asiapcf/09/16/china.tainted.formula/index.html
➤ www.telegraph.co.uk/news/worldnews/asia/china/2827362/Baby-formula-recall-in-China-after-infant-death.html.

REFERENCES

1 Renfrew MJ, Dyson L, Wallace L *et al. The Effectiveness of Public Health Interventions to Promote the Duration of Breastfeeding: systematic review*. London: National Institute for Health and Clinical Excellence; 2005. www.nice.org.uk/page.aspx?o=511622 (accessed 5 October 2009).

2 Tedstone A, Dunce N, Aviles M *et al. Effectiveness of Interventions to Promote Healthy Feeding of Infants Under One Year of Age: review*. London: Health Education Authority; 1998. www.nice.org.uk/page.aspx?o=501963 (accessed 5 October 2009).

3 Fairbank L, O'Meara S, Renfrew MJ *et al.* A systematic review to evaluate the effectiveness of interventions to promote the initiation of breastfeeding. *Health Technol Assess.* 2000; **4**: 1–171.

4 Kelly M, Speller V. *The Health Development Agency and Evidence into Practice*. London: Health Development Agency; 2002.

5 Tarrant M, Dodgson JE, Choi VW. Becoming a role model: the breastfeeding trajectory of Hong Kong women breastfeeding longer than 6 months. *Int J Nurs Stud.* 2004; **41**: 535–46.

6 Boyd JD, Henders D, Lobban G. *Grey Lodge: a century of care and concern*. Undated.

7 European Commission Directorate of Public Health and Risk Assessment. *Protection, Promotion and Support of Breastfeeding in Europe: a blueprint for action*. Luxembourg: European Commission; 2004.

8 Ibid.

9 World Health Organization. *The International Code of Marketing of Breast-Milk Substitutes*. Geneva: World Health Organization; 1981. www.ibfan.org/site2005/Pages/article.php?art_id=52&iui=1 (accessed 5 October 2009).

10 Ibid.

11 Taylor A. Violations of the International Code of Marketing of Breast-Milk Substitutes: prevalence in four countries. *BMJ*. 1998; **316**: 1177–22.

12 UNICEF/WHO. *The UNICEF Baby-Friendly Hospital Initiative: ten steps to successful breastfeeding*. New York: UNICEF; 1992.

13 Ibid.

14 UNICEF. *UNICEF UK Baby-Friendly Initiative: the Seven Point Plan for sustaining breastfeeding in the community*. New York: UNICEF; 2008. www.babyfriendly.org.uk/pdfs/ The_Seven_Point_Plan_September_2008.pdf (accessed 7 October 2009).

15 Malik ANJ, Cutting WAM. Breast feeding: the baby friendly initiative. *BMJ*. 1998; **316**: 1548–9.

16 Moore T, Gauld R, Williams S. *Implementing Baby-Friendly Hospital Initiative Policy: the case of New Zealand public hospitals*. 2007. www.internationalbreastfeedingjournal. com/content/pdf/1746-4358-2-8.pdf (accessed 8 October 2009).

17 Office on Women's Health, US Department of Health and Human Services. *Blueprint for Action on Breastfeeding*. Washington, DC: US Department of Health and Human Services; 2000.

18 American Academy of Pediatrics. Policy statement, breastfeeding and use of human milk. *Pediatrics*. 2005; **115**: 496–506.

19 Directorate of Public Health and Risk Assessment, European Commission. *Protection, Promotion and Support of Breastfeeding in Europe: a blueprint for action*. Luxembourg: European Commission; 2004.

20 World Health Organization. *Global Strategy for Infant and Young Child Feeding*. Geneva: World Health Organization; 2003. http://whqlibdoc.who.int/publications/ 2003/9241562218.pdf (accessed 8 October 2009).

21 World Health Organization. *Effect of Breastfeeding on Mortality among HIV-Infected Women*. Geneva: World Health Organization; 2001.

22 World Health Organization. *Global Strategy for Infant and Young Child Feeding*, op. cit.

23 Ibid.

24 World Health Organization. *Global Immunization Strategy*. 2008. www.who.int/gb/ ebwha/pdf_files/A61/A61_R15-en.pdf (accessed 8 October 2009).

25 Wise J. Companies still breaking milk marketing code. *BMJ*. 1998; **316**: 1111.

26 Taylor A. Violations of the International Code of Marketing of Breast-Milk Substitutes: prevalence in four countries. *BMJ*. 1998; **316**: 1177–22.

27 Watts J. Manufacturers face jail after baby milk kills 50 in China. *Lancet*. 2004; **363**: 1448.

28 Siegel-Itzkovich J. Baby milk manufacturers agree out-of-court settlement. *BMJ*. 2004; **329**: 310.

29 World Health Organization. *Epidemic and Pandemic Alert and Response (EPR): melamine-contaminated powdered infant formula in China*. Geneva: World Health Organization. 2008. www.who.int/csr/don/2008_09_19/en/index.html (accessed 8 October 2009).

30 Ibid.

31 Siegel-Itzkovich J, op cit.

32 Dykes F. Return to breastfeeding: a global health priority. *Br J Midwifery*. 1997; **5**: 344–9.

33 Ibid.

34 Weimer J. *The Economic Benefits of Breastfeeding: a review and analysis*. Washington, DC: Food and Rural Economics Division, USDA Economic Research Service; 2001.

35 Stockdale J. Postmodernity and the new breastfeeding culture. *RCM Midwives J.* 2002; **5**: 256–9.

36 National Conference of State Legislatures. *Breastfeeding Laws.* 2009. www.ncsl.org/programs/health/breast50.htm (accessed 8 October 2009).

CHAPTER 2

The promotion of breastfeeding: a time and a need to change

I just felt kind of resentful actually about how much pressure there was to breastfeed. I decided quite late on that I would give it a go. I was still kind of annoyed that there was all this pressure.[1]

INTRODUCTION

This chapter begins with an exploration of how and why breastfeeding is beneficial, and establishes a link between promotion and professional assessment with the aim of initiation and continuation of breastfeeding. Promoting breastfeeding is thus a professional role and responsibility that requires specialist knowledge and skills. Furthermore, being responsive and proactive in promoting breastfeeding is the responsibility of professionals and should be supported by governments. The chapter goes on to explore how policy and practice in breastfeeding promotion can be challenged, enhanced and developed through the role of the professional, and to examine how changes can be introduced to promote breastfeeding, irrespective of the organisation and community in which the professional works.

The promotion of breastfeeding cannot be separated from the factors that influence a woman's decision about whether or not to breastfeed. It is therefore incumbent on health professionals (nurses, doctors, midwives, health visitors and community nurses) as a group to promote breastfeeding with a sound knowledge and understanding of the complex nature of a woman's decision. At the very least this effort has to balance the marketing policies and practices used by the formula companies when selling baby milk in both the developed and developing worlds.

In many instances, professionals are in a strong position to influence local breastfeeding rates. They have a direct relationship with women who are pregnant and seeking information and support in making decisions about infant feeding. Over the last two decades a substantial body of research evidence has emerged to support the reasons why women should breastfeed. The expectation is that this body of evidence will continue to grow and develop, and that it will become more sophisticated and reliable.

This chapter therefore discusses the psychosocial, economic and political barriers to breastfeeding that practitioners should consider when seeking to promote breastfeeding, particularly in areas where this aim is related to the promotion of health and well-being.

INFANT AND MATERNAL HEALTH

There is a wealth of evidence that breast milk is the most suitable food for babies, and that exclusive breastfeeding has both long-term and short-term health benefits.

The health of the infant

Throughout the centuries, breastfeeding has had support from religious organisations on the basis that it contributes to both the psychological and physical health and well-being of baby and mother. In 1995, His Holiness Pope John Paul II granted a solemn papal audience to the participants of the working group on 'Breastfeeding: Science and Society'. In response to the group report, the Holy Father pronounced on the psychological and physical advantages of breastfeeding to the infant, including protection against disease, and the provision of proper nourishment.

It is known that breastfeeding has preventive properties with regard to illness, and that this could have an impact on healthcare budgets. It has been reported that more than US$ 1 billion are spent each year on the diagnosis and treatment of two diseases that breastfeeding is known to protect against, namely otitis media and gastroenteritis.[2] A report released by the US Department of Agriculture in 2001 calculated that US$ 36 billion would be saved if breastfeeding in the USA increased by 75% of in-hospital mothers, and if 50% of women continued to breastfeed for 6 months.[3] The savings related to only three diseases, namely otitis media, gastroenteritis and necrotising enterocolitis (a gastrointestinal tract disease that is most commonly seen in neonatal infants).

There are a number of specific disease areas for which clear evidence has been gathered. It has been estimated that in Brazil a bottle-fed baby is 14 times more likely to die of diarrhoea and nearly four times more likely to die of a respiratory infection than a baby who has been fed on breast milk.[4] This is not only a problem for the developing world. A Californian study of a relatively affluent, well-educated population found that the rate of diarrhoeal illness in breastfed babies was half that found in bottle-fed infants.[5] A Scottish study also found that the probability of respiratory illness occurring at any time during childhood is significantly reduced if the child is fed breast milk exclusively for the first 15 weeks, and no solid foods are introduced during this time.[6]

There are also long-term benefits in terms of a reduction in the risk of developing atherosclerosis, because breastfeeding is associated with lower cholesterol levels in later life.[7] These findings were supported by an earlier Dutch report which highlighted the protective effects of breastfeeding on adult glucose tolerance, lipid profile, blood pressure and body weight.[8] Interestingly, the subjects in the Dutch study were born between November 1944 and May 1945, which was also a time of severe famine during the German occupation of the Netherlands.

There is also now an established link between breastfeeding and prevention of obesity. Studies from both Scotland[9] and the Czech Republic[10] have found that the overall prevalence of obesity is lower in breastfed children. Similar findings were reported in a study of children from 10 towns in the UK who were born in the affluent 1990s.[11] Although there are many causes of obesity, a German study found that the prevalence of obesity in children who had never been breastfed was 4.5%, compared with 2.8% in breastfed children.[12] This particular study identified a clear dose–response effect for duration of breastfeeding and the prevalence of obesity, as the latter decreased from 3.8% for 2 months of exclusive breastfeeding to 0.8% for more than 12 months of breastfeeding.

The findings with regard to obesity are of particular interest in many developed and developing nations. Developed nations such as the UK, Australia and the USA have immigrant populations who are at high risk due to dietary changes and a genetic predisposition to diseases such as diabetes. Similarly, population groups in developing countries who are relatively wealthy and have a diet with a high content of refined sugars are at high risk of obesity and related diseases such as cancer and diabetes. In developed nations such as the UK and the USA there is also mounting concern about the imminence of obesity epidemics in the younger population as well as the older population. For example, in 2003 in the USA a newspaper reported the death of a 3-year-old child from heart failure, which was attributed to her weight.

Interestingly, a dose–response effect has been associated with breastfeeding in studies that examined the child's Intelligence Quotient (IQ). This has also been reported by several other studies, including studies of children born preterm.[13] The effect is also thought to be linked to neurodevelopment as measured by the developmental milestones during the latter half of infancy.[14] A Danish study has found evidence that the effect persists into adulthood, as when two separate samples of young adults were assessed with two different intelligence tests, a significant positive association was found for the breastfed subjects.[15] New evidence from a large randomised trial following a cohort of children concluded that prolonged exclusive breastfeeding improves children's cognitive development.[16] Attention is also becoming focused on challenges associated with actual reactions and chemicals in breast milk, which may be responsible for the beneficial effects. For example, at its 2004 Annual Meeting, the Pediatric Academic Societies in San Francisco debated whether the possible biological mechanism underlying this protective effect is linked to the protein adiponectin.

Additional studies published towards the end of the twentieth century have collectively summarised the main health benefits of breastfeeding to the baby, some of which extend into adult life. They include a reduction in the following:

➤ gastroenteritis[17-21]

➤ respiratory infections[22-24]

➤ respiratory infections with exclusive breastfeeding to 15 weeks, which persists into childhood[25]

➤ otitis media[26-29]

➤ urinary tract infections[30,31]

➤ allergy, asthma and atopic disease with a family history[32]

➤ insulin-dependent diabetes[33,34]

➤ childhood obesity[35-37]

➤ reduced cholesterol levels[38]

➤ reduced systolic blood pressure.[39,40]

The health of the mother

A meta-analysis of 47 epidemiological studies from 30 countries concluded that the longer the duration of breastfeeding, the higher the level of protection of the mother against breast cancer. It also suggested that the high incidence of breast cancer in the developed world may be partially associated with the fact that many women only breastfeed for a short period of time.[41]

The World Cancer Research Fund (WCRF) published a landmark report in which it presented a comprehensive overview of the links between lifestyle and cancer risk.[42] Scientists suggested that almost one-third of cancer cases could be prevented if the recommendations for cancer prevention were followed. Breastfeeding exclusively for the first 6 months of the infant's life was one of the 10 lifestyle changes recommended for the prevention of cancer.

A link has also been established between breastfeeding and birth spacing. A report published in the *British Journal of Midwifery (BJM)* in 1997 described a review of the anthropological literature in which it was found to be common-place to breastfeed up to the age of 3 or 4 years in some societies.[43] This in turn appeared to create birth spaces of approximately 4 years. In this report a 1988 study is cited which estimated that breastfeeding prevents an average of 4 births per woman in Africa overall, and 6.5 in Bangladesh.[44] In particular this evidence suggests that breastfeeding may provide a degree of contraceptive protection.[45] However, this is not a reliable method for preventing pregnancy. The *BJM* report therefore maintains that formula feeding removes the hormonal influences of breastfeeding, which to a certain extent may be beneficial to women because of the physiological birth-spacing effect.[46]

Different rates of breastfeeding

Despite the compelling evidence for the health consequences of not breastfeeding, in reality it remains difficult for some women to choose to breastfeed. Only 2% of Swedish babies are never breastfed, compared with 29% of babies in the UK.[47] It is estimated that only around 50% of babies in the Western world are breastfed at 6 weeks. In the UK, the percentage of women who start to breastfeed fell from 70% in the 1970s to 60% in the 1990s.[48] The duration of breastfeeding also varies. Around 80% of Egyptian mothers breastfeed for at least 6 months, and 40% for 15–18 months.[49] In comparison, 64% of American mothers breastfeed in hospital, and only 29% are still breastfeeding 6 months later.[50] In Scotland, around 50% of new mothers initiate breastfeeding, yet Scotland has the lowest rate of breastfeeding in the UK, and many observers blame social attitudes to breastfeeding for this situation.[51]

The attitudes that women encounter and the pressures that they are under in developed countries in the twenty-first century create their own barriers. Zimmerman and Guttman sought the views of both breastfeeding mothers and formula-feeding mothers and found that both agreed that breastfeeding was better for the baby.[52] However, it appears from this study that knowing this is not enough to persuade mothers to start and then continue to breastfeed. The convenience factors and involvement of others in feeding the baby, particularly fathers, were important considerations when deciding whether or not to breastfeed. Both groups in the study rated formula feeding as better because it allowed others to help with infant care, enabling the mother to have more control over her time and greater freedom. Other studies have also highlighted the fact that formula feeding provides greater opportunities for fathers to feed the baby.[53]

AMBIGUITY AND CONTROVERSY IN THE PUBLIC AND POLITICAL ARENA

Public support

In some countries, negative or ambivalent attitudes among the general public towards breastfeeding may be rooted in the ambiguity that surrounds the function of the breast as a natural means of feeding offspring and as a focus that incites sexual and erotic emotions. Government action can help to drive change in values and attitudes over time, and thus to shape attitudes to health and healthy living within society. For example, in the early 1990s, Florida was the only state in the USA with legislation that guaranteed a mother's right to breastfeed in public without being arrested for indecent exposure.[54]

Two political developments in the UK demonstrate positive government action, but at the same time reflect the degree of ambiguity and confusion that may exist in a society. A Scottish Parliamentary Bill that was introduced in 2004 made it an offence to stop a mother breastfeeding in public. This policy change came after reports of nursing mothers being asked to leave dentists' and doctors' waiting rooms, restaurants, shopping centres and buses.[55]

At the same time as this legislation was passed, UK censors banned the fleeting image of an exposed nipple in an advertisement promoting voting in the 2004 European Union elections as being too sexual. A similar example of ambiguity can be found in the USA, where an organisation that publicly endorses breastfeeding also distributes vouchers for formula foods under the US Women, Infants and Children (WIC) programme. Riordan and Gill-Hopple commented on the problems that health professionals had with WIC promoting breastfeeding but at the same time giving out formula infant milk.[56]

Thus the WIC programme seems to be simultaneously promoting and supporting breastfeeding and giving formula manufacturers direct access to women. In fact it is selling formula products to the very population that would gain considerable health benefits if they chose to breastfeed. Riordan and Gill-Hopple also noted that Cambodian women in Dallas were understood to talk about the WIC office as the place where they could be given formula feed. This helps to explain the finding that women immigrants in the USA are more likely to choose formula feeding over breastfeeding the longer they live in the USA, even if their country of origin is one where breastfeeding rates are high.[57]

In the UK, infant formula milk was sold in community health centres as part of the welfare foods system. The public could therefore buy infant formula at a price which was usually significantly lower than that in the supermarket. The removal of infant formula sales as part of the Healthy Start initiative took place in November 2006. The beneficiaries of the Healthy Start initiative receive vouchers which are reimbursed at participating retailers, mainly the major supermarket chains and shops that sell fruit, vegetables, milk and infant formula. The ultimate effect of this change was to move the advertising and consequent conflicting messages from the community health centres into the retail sector.

Further information on the Healthy Start initiative can be found on their website (www.healthystart.nhs.uk).

Family support

The type of social environment in which a woman lives and the quality of family support that she receives have been found to have a direct effect on her decision as to whether to breastfeed. A Scottish study found that breastfeeding mothers are more likely to be married or living with a partner, to be owners of their homes, and to smoke less than bottle-feeding mothers.[58] Furthermore, the mothers in this study who breastfed were more likely to have decided on the infant feeding method before conception, were more likely to have attended parentcraft classes, were more often from a higher social class, were older and had a longer duration of higher education.

However, ambivalence and ambiguity may exist at the family level. Although some partners find lactating breasts sexually attractive during lovemaking, others do not, and this has the potential to create a barrier to the woman initiating and/or continuing breastfeeding, depending on the circumstances. Other forces may also be operating, such as a woman deriving sexual pleasure from breastfeeding, which reduces her desire to resume a sexual relationship with her partner.[59] Conversely, breastfeeding can be painful and stressful, and may be regarded as potentially excluding the mother from social activities. The high prolactin levels and low oestrogen levels of the lactating mother can also reduce her libido.[60,61]

Psychological factors may also affect the attitude of the woman's partner. For example, it has been suggested that some men may subconsciously revisit sibling rivalry, harking back to memories of jealousy when a younger brother or sister was being breastfed, and a time when they were competing with the infant for the breast or the mother's attention.

On the other hand, many fathers enjoy the breastfeeding months and derive much pleasure and joy from the experience. Breastfeeding does not negate opportunities for fathers to feed the baby breast milk and to share in the experience of feeding the baby. If this is the aim, this practice should be established as early as possible. It will involve the mother learning how to express breast milk, and as breast milk is relatively fast flowing, a bottle with a large-holed teat or a feeding cup should be used to feed the baby. Feeding a baby breast milk from a bottle or cup may be a particular priority for a woman, and if so, this practice should be established as early as possible.[62,63]

Lifestyle and convenience

The women and babies who have the most to gain from breastfeeding are those who are socially deprived, and it is this group that has the lowest uptake of breastfeeding and possibly presents the greatest challenge.[64] Ironically, low income and full-time employment are juxtaposed as barriers, and other factors are also relevant, including the following:

➤ embarrassment about the act of breastfeeding and fear of exposure of the breast remain major challenges in relation to health promotion.[65-67]
➤ women who have experienced breastfeeding problems[68]
➤ lack of a supportive partner[69]
➤ multiparous women who have not breastfed previously[70,71]
➤ type of delivery and whether a general anaesthetic has been administered[72-74]
➤ low-birthweight babies.[75]

It is known that in developed countries the younger the mother is, the less likely she is to breastfeed.[76,77] Adolescent mothers are therefore likely to present a particular challenge in terms of breaking down existing barriers to breastfeeding. A study of 25 African-American adolescent mothers in Florida during 1999–2000 found that adolescent mothers do not have the characteristics that are known to be associated with breastfeeding continuation, such as older age, higher level of education, being married or living with a partner, and higher income.[78] It was also noted that adolescent mothers are particularly concerned about body image issues raised by breastfeeding.

Practice expert

It is important to acknowledge that groups should not be stereotyped as likely to show a set of predictable behaviours. The following account demonstrates how one teenage mother described her motivation to breastfeed.

Vignette: View of a teenager

'I just thought of the health benefits, that was high priority for me. I wanted the children to have the best, but I think I was also driven by stereotyping of teenage mothers. I was 19 when I had Mark, and I think that played a big aspect. I wanted to show society that just because I'm a young mum it doesn't mean to say I'm not a good mum and that I don't want the best for my children. I was at a park with the kids and there were a lot of children playing. Behind me there was a middle-class couple discussing the local teenage pregnancy rate and blabbing about teenage pregnancies. So I started to breastfeed as a protest to their attitude.'

Reflect

Linked to the fact that this teenager was well informed, what are the views and perceptions of teenagers generally? What types of specific support may be given to young mothers to breastfeed?

In all groups there may be a misinformed value set that needs to be identified, such as believing that bottle feeding is best because bottle-fed babies gain weight faster and this is associated with health.[79]

Employment law and working practices

In both the developed and developing worlds, women work outside the home and need to manage the competing demands of work and infant feeding. Economic necessity is often the driver for women returning to work before their baby is 6 months of age. The reality of the situation is that in many countries women are compelled by law to return to work, otherwise they may risk losing their job.

Some workplaces, including major companies in Europe and the USA, proactively create opportunities for mothers to breastfeed by providing on-site crèches and 'time out' for women to breastfeed and express milk. Other countries, such as Norway, provide longer maternity (and paternity) leave to enable the child to breastfeed for the optimal first 6 months.[80] In Norway this policy has had the effect of dramatically increasing breastfeeding rates, with initiation rates of breastfeeding of 98% at hospital discharge, and 75% of women continuing to breastfeed after 6 months.[81]

Practice expert

For some mothers, the practicalities of coping with a busy work, family and/or social life take precedence when deciding whether or not to breastfeed. In these circumstances, employment law and practices are particularly relevant, as is professional help to establish a suitable compromise to enable breastfeeding.

Vignette: Getting back to work

'I don't think I wanted to breastfeed at all at the time. I thought "If I breastfeed then I'm never going to be able to leave him." It was my first baby and I was fully expecting it just to be pretty much exactly as it was before I actually had him. I was going to go back to work, and I had friends and family and a little bit of childcare sorted out. I was going to go back to full-time work, and even though it wouldn't pay very well, at least it would get me out of the house.'

Reflect

What sort of effective and accurate information about employees' rights can be offered? What real-life examples of and practical advice about returning to work while continuing to breastfeed can be provided?

The situation in Norway demonstrates that the political climate and political action can have a substantial impact in promoting breastfeeding and raising breastfeeding rates. For example, in the climate of 'workfare not welfare', women in the USA who need the help of the Supplemental Food Program under WIC are encouraged to look for work and to use day care for their infants.[82] Since many of these women will be in the adolescent category, and given the prevailing evidence that adolescent mothers and their babies benefit from breastfeeding, such policies may have the unintentional effect of discouraging young women from breastfeeding.

INTRINSIC MATERNAL BEHAVIOUR
Self-efficacy

If we are truly to embrace the need to increase support for breastfeeding, there must be an understanding of the factors that influence and determine the behaviours of breastfeeding women. The concept of self-efficacy is closely related to the level of an individual's self-confidence. Self-efficacy is an inner belief in one's ability to achieve a task.[83] Maternal self-confidence and belief in one's ability to breastfeed are considered to be modifiable variables.[84] In two studies, Bandura identified that if an individual has low self-efficacy, they will avoid tasks and give up quickly.[85,86] When deciding whether to breastfeed, a woman's self-efficacy is a highly significant factor, as it may have a strong positive influence on her decision and potential ability to breastfeed.[87]

Perceptions of and levels of self-efficacy have a significant influence on how an individual judges their abilities to perform certain behaviours, and greatly influence the choice of and persistence with certain behaviours. Highly efficacious people are more likely to master tasks and to persevere when faced with problems, but only if they believe that the task will result in a certain positive outcome.

A study of the psychosocial factors that influence breastfeeding found maternal confidence to be one of the most significant variables affecting duration of breastfeeding.[88] Similarly, Buxton et al. found that 27% of women with low maternal confidence in the prenatal period discontinued breastfeeding in the first postpartum week, compared with only 5% of highly confident women.[89]

A breastfeeding self-efficacy measurement tool has been developed[90] based on Bandura's *theory of social learning*.[91] The theoretical underpinning of the tool is that self-efficacy is central to social learning and is considered to be a dynamic cognitive process, associated with the ability of an individual to self-assess their ability to perform a certain behaviour.

Measuring self-efficacy

Blythe *et al.* also showed that antenatal and 1-week postpartum self-efficacy scores correlated significantly with breastfeeding outcomes at 1 week and 4 months.[92] Mothers with a high self-efficacy score were more likely to be breastfeeding and doing so exclusively at 1 week and 4 months than those who had low breastfeeding self-efficacy scores. Dennis and Faux have suggested that the ability to be efficacious is a predictor of choice and the degree of effort that a woman will invest in establishing breastfeeding.[93] The use of the Dennis and Faux tool or a similar assessment instrument may increase a professional's ability to refine and tune information giving to meet individual needs, and considerably enhance the potential to promote breastfeeding. It has been suggested that using this tool to assess a woman's level of self-efficacy will predict:

➤ whether a mother chooses to breastfeed or bottle feed
➤ how much effort she will expend on breastfeeding
➤ whether she will have self-enhancing or self-defeating thought patterns
➤ how she will respond emotionally to breastfeeding difficulties.

Practice expert

The experiences that women have with breastfeeding a first baby will influence the investment and effort that they put into breastfeeding a second baby. Self-efficacy is also a consideration, as this is a factor that is known to determine whether a woman will continue or stop breastfeeding. The burning question is whether the degree of success or failure weakens or strengthens a woman's resolve to breastfeed a second child.

Vignette: Past experience influences behaviour

'I didn't try as hard with J because I didn't want to go through all this upset again if he didn't go for it straight away. I never really gave it much of a chance, I must admit. They were doing it for me – trying to get it into her mouth and stuff – but she just wasn't having it. As I said she got a couple of breastfeeds, but when I got home I thought I've got to do this myself, there's nobody here to help me, and I just went on to bottles.'

Reflect

Breastfeeding appeared to be a passive experience for this mother, and she clearly had no expectation of receiving reliable continuous support. Do self-efficacy and continuous support go together hand in hand? What behaviours and factors demonstrate self-efficacy or lack of confidence? How can these factors be assessed by the professional so that they can judge the woman's level of self-efficacy? Finally, what strategies could be adopted by the professional to increase the woman's self-efficacy?

Dennis and Faux further suggest that gaining and building confidence in breast-feeding are associated with three specific experiences:[94]

➤ performance accomplishments (e.g. previously breastfed baby)
➤ vicarious experience (e.g. watching other women successfully breastfeeding)
➤ verbal persuasion (e.g. factual information, encouragement from influential others such as family, friends and professionals).

Practice expert

Low self-efficacy will have a negative effect on a woman's ability to make decisions and choices about breastfeeding. It will also affect her ability to persevere and her confidence in managing the practicalities of breastfeeding. These issues are raised in the account below.

Vignette: Previous difficulties will have a negative influence

'Probably I decided to bottle feed because I hadn't made any decisions while I was pregnant. I had tried when I had my first baby, C, and it wasn't a great experience, so I think I was probably going into it negatively. When I had my second baby, R, I wasn't working, but this time I had recently been promoted at work. I started by thinking "If I am out of the house for 24 hours at a time, how do I manage breastfeeding?" I think all of these things were in my mind, and I wasn't able to find a way to solve it.'

Reflect

How important is it, in terms of policy, practice and service delivery, to assume that breastfeeding women have specific needs? Could breastfeeding rates possibly be increased substantially if this fact was taken into consideration in service development and delivery?

A self-efficacy tool can be used with accompanying strategies that aim to improve the confidence of new mothers in their ability both to breastfeed and to persevere in establishing breastfeeding when difficulties are encountered.[95] Consideration should be given to the competence of healthcare professionals in the use of self-efficacy tools and associated strategies, and how these can be integrated effectively into educational and health approaches to breastfeeding.

The concept of 'embodied knowledge'

The link between knowledge exposure and attitude formation is substantiated by a study which identified that breastfeeding mothers regarded breastfeeding as more convenient, whereas formula-feeding mothers considered bottle feeding to be more convenient.[96] Hoddinott and Pill conducted a study on attitude formation in first-time mothers living in the East End of London.[97] Using semi-structured interviews, this study found that the knowledge and experience gained by close exposure to and observation of the breastfeeding experiences of others, during what can be considered an informative period, represented 'embodied knowledge' of breastfeeding. A key point that emerged from the study was that women who observed other women, friends or relatives breastfeeding successfully were more likely to start breastfeeding their own children, and to continue to breastfeed successfully.

Practice expert

There is evidence that breastfeeding rates can be increased in first-time mothers if they actually see for themselves the positive benefits to be gained from breastfeeding. The best role models for this are family and relevant others.

Vignette: Seeing is believing

'A lot of people think it's better breastfeeding, but I'd rather bottle feed. When I get pregnant with the next one, I'm going to try breastfeeding. My friend and my cousin, they are all breastfeeding, and their babies seem a lot better. My friend has breastfed her little boy for a month and he feeds much better.'

Reflect

What strategies might professionals use in situations where women do not have the benefit of role models for breastfeeding in their family or social circle?

Role modelling is linked directly to an individual's value system and attitudes. It has also been found that the grandmother's attitude, particularly the attitude of the maternal grandmother, is very influential.[98,99] The influence of the partner and family in the decision as to whether or not to breastfeed was also highlighted in an American study in an urban, predominantly African-American population.[100] African-American women have a lower rate of breastfeeding than Caucasian Americans and Hispanic Americans, and a study of African-American women at two US military healthcare clinics emphasised the need for healthcare workers to promote breastfeeding.[101]

A Scottish study also found similar results, and concluded that the partner's experience and attitude were crucial in determining whether or not to breastfeed. This study advocated that breastfeeding should be included in personal and social development classes in Scottish primary schools, so that the attitudes of both boys and girls towards breastfeeding are shaped at an early stage.[102]

The concept of 'embodied knowledge' cannot be separated from that of peer influence. They are in all respects two sides of the same coin. In the UK, peer-group influence among teenage parents has been associated with deterring young women from breastfeeding.[103] A study of Texan teenage mothers in the late 1990s found that 35% of them planned to breastfeed.[104] Of these individuals, a minority were black women, compared with a majority of Mexican American mothers and a smaller but similar proportion of Caucasian women. Interestingly, of these three cultural groups, black women were least likely to have received encouragement to breastfeed from a healthcare provider, partner, parent or friend. In this case the lack of both a role model and professional support may have resulted in the lower breastfeeding rates.

A recent Canadian study[105] found peer support to be even more important than advice from health professionals. Another study in this area demonstrates the crucial influence of role modelling and peer support on an individual's value set, attitude and behaviour.[106] This is a particularly important finding in geographical areas and social groupings where bottle feeding is the norm, and it provides an insight into how decisions to bottle feed are perpetuated over time, through social customs and habits.

PROFESSIONAL KNOWLEDGE AND COMPETENCE
Informed choice

A woman's decision to breastfeed is thus a complex process that involves multiple variables relating to the mother, the baby, the family and the wider social and political environment. Changing current practices requires professionals to question and analyse the complex social and political structures in which contemporary women operate. An important consideration is that as global and national policy moves to support breastfeeding, women who do not choose to breastfeed may naturally feel (or be made to feel) guilty.[107] This consideration highlights the necessity for monitoring the quality of decision-making processes that can be accessed by professionals who are involved in information giving.

The aim of information giving is to enable women to make well-informed individual decisions about infant feeding, and ultimately for them to choose a feeding method that best suits their particular circumstances, and to be comfortable with whatever method they decide to adopt. It is fundamental to this process that the healthcare professional provides objective, accurate and up-to-date information, and that when appropriate they raise awareness of the social and political factors that affect decisions to breastfeed.

Practice expert

Strategies to promote breastfeeding must be well thought through, and should be client or woman centred. A 'one size fits all' approach is unlikely to be successful, and may even be counter-productive.

Vignette: It's not just what you say, but how you say it

'I wasn't sure if I was going to breastfeed at all. I did feel kind of resentful that I might have pressure. I called the midwives the breastfeeding Gestapo. Basically every time I went to see the midwife, I think they had a student who had done a little display that was just above the desk so all the expectant mothers would come in and sit in the chair facing this display about how important breastfeeding was. I just felt kind of resentful actually about how much pressure there was to breastfeed. I decided quite late on that I would give it a go. I was still kind of annoyed that there was all this pressure. In the end I thought I would give it a go.'

Reflect

This mother's description of breastfeeding promotion during pregnancy includes thought-provoking comments about her experience. It is important for healthcare professionals to stop and listen to the views of the women whom they serve.

Professional assessment of social factors

When discussing breastfeeding, professionals are in an ethical, political and social relationship with a woman. What information is communicated and the way in which this is done will determine whether an informed choice can be made. Information giving on the part of the professional, and informed choice on the part of the woman, are therefore at the heart of the decision-making process, which is itself affected by a number of related issues, including:

- the research rigour and knowledge base of the professional
- the amount of time allocated to information giving
- the creation of a range of opportunities for communicating information
- the consistency of information that is provided
- whether information is up to date
- the frequency with which information is provided.

Practice expert

Breastfeeding promotion can be perceived by women as preaching rather than as information giving. However, promotion goes beyond information giving to include an element of persuasion. The act of persuasion in a healthcare context is in turn dependent on listening to the views and concerns of service users and dealing with the issues that emerge from this dialogue. The challenge for the professional in promoting breastfeeding is to find the time and opportunity to listen to women and to use the right strategies during promotion sessions, such as providing a safe environment and encouraging and supporting women to 'speak up' and 'speak out.'

Vignette: How women perceive and receive promotion
'It's finding a way to talk to people so that they'll be receptive, too, and having that information there for them without shoving it down their throats.'

Reflect
How can the professional promote breastfeeding with a human face and without seeming to 'preach' to the woman?

Information management
In societies where giving information about breastfeeding involves challenging prevailing social norms, there will be a need for health professionals to create new approaches, systems and structures and a range of opportunities to support the information-giving process. Incorporated in these systems there should be a range of flexible opportunities, designed for and integrated throughout the whole of pregnancy, to discuss breastfeeding both individually and in groups. It must be recognised by managers and practitioners alike that both time commitment and creative approaches are required in order to deal with the complexity of factors relating to individual decisions to breastfeed, and to help and support women as they untangle issues in the context of their individual social and psychological networks and specific personal circumstances. Information giving alone is therefore a completely inadequate strategy. It must be supported by robust systems where information is linked to professional values and goals such as currency, convenience, creativity, caring, continuity and consistency.

Practice expert
There can be a large gap between intention and effect. The professional needs to be constantly aware of this relationship.

Vignette: Empowering through promotion
'People like health visitors need to give you the choice rather than say you must breastfeed because it is best for the baby. It would stop mothers saying "I don't want to breastfeed" or "I was thinking about breastfeeding." I think if they stopped pushing it on mothers and let them make their own decisions it would be a lot better.'

> **Reflect**
> It is not always easy for the professional to get the balance right. When aiming to promote breastfeeding, how necessary is individual assessment and building a relationship between the woman and the professional over time?

Using a blend of approaches to information giving

The most effective professional systems have in place a blend of different approaches to information giving, with information being delivered by different media and different individuals, and they monitor the effect of these on breast-feeding continuation rates. Information should be delivered in a form that is most appropriate to the needs and wants of your local population. For example, during pregnancy, interactive groups and culture-specific sessions have been shown to have a positive effect on the duration of breastfeeding.[108] Breastfeeding workshops or group sessions demonstrating positioning and attachment have also shown longer-term positive results.[109] The main principles of information giving are as follows:

- consistency of information between and among professionals
- all information being accurate and up to date
- frequent review of information used
- evaluation of the effectiveness of information given
- use of more than one individual or format to provide the same information
- repetition of the same information several times using different individuals and different formats
- use of a range of different formats to convey the same message (e.g. verbal, written, poster, group session, and one-to-one session).

The effect of information delivery systems should be evaluated. The following 10 criteria provide guidance on how to measure the quality of information giving. It should be:

- consistent over time, between different people and different formats
- up to date, reflecting current thinking and evidence
- evidence based as far as possible
- delivered with due consideration to taking time and effort to explain thoroughly any grey and controversial areas of evidence
- delivered at the right time, by the right person and at the right level
- meaningful to the personal needs and wants of the woman
- meaningful to the personal needs and wants of the baby
- meaningful to the family context of the individual
- meaningful to the social and cultural context of the individual
- delivered in different forms.

Evidence base for practice

The general increasing interest in breastfeeding is an interesting and contemporary phenomenon that is juxtaposed with commitment by the healthcare professions to evidence-based practice. From the perspective of the professional, these two trends are complementary, and are mutually supportive of efforts to ensure that both policy making and professional practice are developed and implemented from a rigorous research base.

A range of issues associated with breaking down the barriers to breastfeeding are directly related to professional practice. These issues are interrelated and present the professional with a kaleidoscope of politico-economic and psychosocial challenges in promoting breastfeeding. Evidence exists which suggests that a wide range of psychosocial factors can act as barriers and influence women against choosing to breastfeed.[110-116] Furthermore, there are also barriers associated with groups in society who have specific social and economic needs. These needs are likely to influence the willingness and ability of mothers to breastfeed. For example, as has already been noted, it is recognised that women who live in the most disadvantaged areas and who are on low income are less likely to breastfeed.

Research rigour in breastfeeding studies and translating research evidence into practice has been high on the agenda of the healthcare professions for the last quarter of a century. Early research involving 'before and after' studies of breastfeeding rates,[117] and a decade later studies of high-school girls' attitudes towards breastfeeding,[118] have been criticised for lack of concurrent controls.[119] Almost a generation later the same criticism remains, specifically with regard to the dearth of randomised or non-randomised controlled trials of breastfeeding.[120]

A review by Fairbank *et al.* brought specific attention to bear on the research methods of multi-faceted intervention studies, which used 'before and after' methods to evaluate certain educational, health and peer support factors and some forms of media activity.[121] Particular concerns were raised about external factors that were present prior to or during the evaluations, and which may have adversely affected the findings.

This is an important criticism. Although breastfeeding per se is very difficult to study using randomised controlled trials (RCTs), the effects of interventions can be studied. As the amount of research evidence that can be drawn upon increases, attention is focused on the level of professional competence and confidence in accessing research literature, assessing its rigour and determining its relevance to breastfeeding practices and policy. This will be discussed in more detail in Chapter 6.

In the UK, the major systematic review conducted by Renfrew *et al.* into the effectiveness of public health interventions to promote breastfeeding concluded that a move towards evidence-based care will require major changes in the systems which are currently operating, and that changes in attitudes towards breastfeeding will also be required, from senior level to grassroots level.[122]

The publication of that review in 2005 stimulated national debate about the lack of research evidence available from populations in the UK.[123] This has resulted in an awareness of effective and ineffective interventions, encouraging and promoting changes in practice by healthcare professionals. In addition, such publications have enabled the design of bespoke interventions that are responsive to local population needs.

In summary, a wealth of literature has been published which has reviewed the research evidence and provided guidance on the most effective interventions to support the initiation and continuation of breastfeeding.[124-127] The interventions that were shown to be effective included:

➤ peer support
➤ professional support
➤ education
➤ education and professional support
➤ education and peer support
➤ professional training
➤ hospital practices
➤ multisectoral interventions
➤ media programmes.

Following on from this work, an 'Evidence into Practice' briefing was published in 2006, which presented a number of evidence-based actions for promoting the initiation and continuation of breastfeeding, with a focus on vulnerable groups, whose breastfeeding rates are lowest.[128] The rationale for this publication stemmed from identified gaps in criteria for systematic reviews, which may then not include some reliable and rigorous studies. From these identified studies, evidence-based actions were generated, which provided the basis for a national consultation with practitioners about experiences and practice. The overarching aim was to generate an approach that would work in real practice in terms of improving breastfeeding rates in England. Full methodological details of the development of the evidence base are provided in the technical report, which is available on request from the National Institute for Health and Clinical Excellence (NICE).[129]

Eight overarching evidence-based actions were recommended, highlighting the need for changes to the way in which services were provided.

1 The UK UNICEF Baby-Friendly Initiative (BFI) practice standards should be implemented in the maternity and community services.
2 A mixture of education and/or support programmes should be delivered by healthcare professionals and peers during pregnancy, tailored to local population needs.
3 Changes to policy and practice within the community and hospital settings should be implemented for helping with positioning and attachment, baby-led feeding, supportive encouragement and management of 'insufficient milk.'

4 Baby-led feeding and rooming in should be encouraged, and unnecessary supplementing of feeding with infant formula, giving discharge packs to mothers, and advertising formula products both in hospital and in the community should be avoided.
5 Complementary telephone peer support should be provided to support continuation of breastfeeding.
6 Breastfeeding education and support from one professional should be targeted at women on low incomes to increase the rates of exclusive breastfeeding.
7 One-to-one needs-based breastfeeding education in the antenatal period, combined with postnatal support through the first year, should be available to increase intention and initiation rates and duration.
8 Media programmes should be developed to target the teenage population.

The healthcare professional can utilise the information provided as evidence-based actions at both individual and community levels, to provide women with information to enable them to make an informed decision about breastfeeding.

Reflect
- Appraise language and communication approaches. Are they discursive or dictatorial in approach?
- How can the UK UNICEF Baby-Friendly Initiative be supported locally?
- Appraise practice against the UK UNICEF Baby-Friendly Initiative.
- Identify the training and support available locally to help with breastfeeding support.
- Consider how local peer support and volunteering opportunities can be assisted.
- Encourage women to make contact with others who are breastfeeding.
- Explore local interventions which have been designed specifically to meet the needs of vulnerable and disadvantaged groups, and make referrals to these services.

CONCLUSION

There is clear evidence of the benefits of breastfeeding to baby and mother, although it is also clear that not all women may wish to breastfeed. There also appear to be large economic benefits to be gained from increasing breastfeeding rates. Informed decision making is an ethical prerogative, while an acceptable target for strategic planners is to support a service to help 75% of women to breastfeed. The emphasis in this chapter has been on promotion of breastfeeding. The issue of continuity of support is dealt with in Chapters 3 and 4.

This chapter suggests that the promotion of breastfeeding should be undertaken by all healthcare professionals who are in contact with pregnant mothers or new families. Consider how small changes can make a real difference to women and their families. A fundamental premise is that effective promotion has the potential to directly influence local and national breastfeeding rates. However, success is predicated on women having continuous support to initiate and continue breastfeeding. These aspects are also dealt with in Chapters 3 and 4.

ANALYSING PRACTICE TO EFFECT CHANGE: A MODEL FOR IMPROVEMENT

The application of improvement methodology to aid the analysis of practice and in turn develop an improvement plan has been used very successfully across many countries. This book is not designed to provide a comprehensive overview of health service improvement, but it does provide some examples of application and how to utilise this methodology in practical terms. For more detailed information, visit the Institute for Healthcare Improvement (IHI) website (www.ihi.org) or consult local improvement and modernisation departments.

A two-part model
Part 1: Enquiry
This involves asking three fundamental questions about current practice.
1 What are we trying to accomplish?
2 How will we know that a change is an improvement?
3 What changes can we make that will result in improvement?

Part 2: Plan–do–study–act (PDSA)
PDSA provides a systematic and cyclic method for testing and implementing changes in real work settings. The PDSA cycle guides the test of change to determine whether the change is in effect an improvement.

Having in place an Improvement Team
Underpinning this cyclic process and application is the appointment of an Improvement Team, which is responsible for leading and managing change by:
➤ setting aims
➤ selecting changes
➤ testing changes
➤ implementing changes
➤ spreading changes.

Applying the improvement model
When considering any changes necessary, and to help to ascertain whether the change has been an improvement, there are nine distinct areas where consideration must be given to the improvement process (although they may not all be relevant for every proposed change).

➤ Eliminate waste.
➤ Improve workflow.
➤ Optimise the inventory.
➤ Change the work environment.
➤ The producer–customer interface.
➤ Manage time.
➤ Focus on variation.
➤ Error-proofing
➤ Focus on the product or service.

Example

Consider the challenges of providing information to pregnant women to help them to make informed decisions about feeding choices, applying the improvement methodology to antenatal preparation for breastfeeding.

➤ The Improvement Team poses the questions in order to fully understand the issues. Integral to this approach are engagement and consultation with the service delivery staff and service users. Table 2.1 shows the proposed change in relation to the improvement areas listed above.

The same headings and approaches can be used to look at different issues, such as how information is provided to women at booking clinic and subsequent points of contact, in order to ensure that all opportunities and contacts during pregnancy are utilised to optimal effect.

FURTHER READING

The MIDIRS website (www.infochoice.org) provides a range of information for healthcare professionals and women on making an informed choice about breastfeeding.

TABLE 2.1 Applying the improvement model

What are we trying to accomplish?	How will we know that a change is an improvement?	What changes can we make that will result in an improvement?
Complete booking appointment for all pregnant women within 1 hour (change to be achieved within 12 months).	Eliminate waste. Reduce time spent booking pregnant women into maternity services.	Measure the time taken to book pregnant women. Ask women about their experience of booking clinic. Ask staff about their experience of booking clinic process. Involve improvement team in 'hunches' for change. PDSA small tests of change (e.g. Can women complete their own booking record prior to clinic appointment? Will this save time?) Complete PDSA record. Plan spread of change.
	Improve workflow. Optimise clinic times and number of women seen by a midwife.	Establish location of booking clinics and times. Are clinics in the right place? Are clinics held at the right time? Is time wasted travelling to multiple city venues? Can the number of venues be reduced? Ask service users whether location is right for them. Review other family-friendly premises.
	Manage time. Optimise and utilise venues available for service.	PDSA alternative venue. Measure service user satisfaction. Review staff output. PDSA clinic venues.

What are we trying to accomplish?	How will we know that a change is an improvement?	What changes can we make that will result in an improvement?
	Optimise the inventory. Effective delivery of care and information to prepare breastfeeding women.	Are staff utilised effectively at booking clinics? Are clinics in the right location?
	Change the work environment. Staff are competent in communication skills and motivational interviewing.	Undertake training needs analysis. Explore health-improvement-specific collaborative training. Identify key operational personnel to attend training. PDSA implementation of agreed changes to booking process.
	Producer–customer interface. Effective and meaningful community engagement to assist in service improvement to meet local needs.	How can health services communicate in the right way with local service users? Ask women for their views about clinic environment, satisfaction, process waiting times. Seek solutions from service users. Use storyboards to publicise changes being implemented in clinic. Encourage feedback.
	Focus on variation. Alternative pathways and process systems established to meet the needs of specific groups.	Develop time variables for different categories of pregnancy. Develop booking pathways and referrals. Find and prevent bottlenecks.

TABLE 2.2 Applying the improvement model to different issues

What are we trying to accomplish?	How will we know that a change is an improvement?	What changes can we make that will result in improvement?
Ensure completion of antenatal breastfeeding checklist by providing information and the opportunity to discuss breastfeeding at all antenatal clinic appointments within 12 months.		

REFERENCES

1 Dalzell J. *Exploring the infant feeding experiences of low-income mothers and the support offered by health professionals involved in their care: a qualitative study.* University of Dundee; 2007. Unpublished.

2 Dewey KG, Heinig J, Nommsen-Rivers LA. Differences in morbidity between breast-fed and formula-fed infants. *J Pediatr.* 1995; **126**: 696–702.

3 Weimer J. *The Economic Benefits of Breastfeeding: a review and analysis.* Washington, DC: Food and Rural Economics Division, USDA Economic Research Service; 2001.

4 Victora CG, Smith PG, Vaughan JP *et al.* Evidence for protection by breast-feeding against infant deaths from infectious diseases in Brazil. *Lancet.* 1987; **330**: 319–22.

5 Dewey KG, Heinig J, Nommsen-Rivers LA, op. cit.

6 Wilson A, Forsyth SA, Greene SA *et al.* Relation of infant feeding to childhood health: seven-year follow-up of cohort of children in Dundee infant feeding study. *BMJ.* 1998; **3**: 21–5.

7 Singhal A, Cole TJ, Fewtrell M *et al.* Breastmilk feeding and lipoprotein profile in adolescents born preterm: follow-up of a prospective randomised study. *Lancet.* 2004; **363**: 1571–8.

8 Ravellie ACJ, van der Meulen JHP, Osmond C *et al.* Infant feeding and adult glucose tolerance, lipid profile, blood pressure and obesity. *Arch Dis Child.* 2000; **82**: 248–52.

9 Armstrong J, Reilly J, Child Health Information Team. Breastfeeding and lowering the risk of childhood obesity. *Lancet.* 2002; **359**: 2003–4.

10 Toschke AM, Vignerova J, Lhotaka L *et al.* Overweight and obesity in 6- to 14-year-old Czech children in 1991: protective effect of breastfeeding. *J Pediatr.* 2002; **141**: 764–9.

11 Owen CG, Whincup PH, Odoki K *et al.* Infant feeding and blood cholesterol: a study in adolescents and a systematic review. *Pediatrics.* 2002; **110**: 597–608.

12 von Kries R, Koletzko B, Sauerwald T *et al.* Breastfeeding and obesity: cross-sectional study. *BMJ.* 1999; **319**: 147–50.

13 Lucas A, Morley R, Cole TJ *et al.* Breast milk and subsequent intelligence quotient in children born preterm. *Lancet.* 1992; **339**: 261–4.

14 Ibid.

15 Mortensen EL, Michaelsen KF, Sanders SA *et al*. The association between duration of breastfeeding and adult intelligence. *JAMA*. 2002; **287**: 2365–71.

16 Kramer MS, Guo T, Platt RW *et al*. Breastfeeding and infant growth: biology or bias? *Pediatrics*. 2002; **110**: 343–7.

17 Victora *et al.*, op. cit.

18 Howie PW, Forsyth JS, Ogston SA *et al*. Protective effect of breastfeeding against infection. *BMJ*. 1990; **300**: 11–16.

19 Popkin BM, Adair L, Akin JS *et al*. Breastfeeding and diarrheal morbidity. *Pediatrics*. 1990; **86**: 874–82.

20 Kramer MS, Guo T, Platt RW *et al*. Infant growth and health outcomes associated with 3 compared with 6 months of exclusive breastfeeding. *Am J Clin Nutr*. 2003; **78**: 291–5.

21 Beaudry M, Dufour R, Marcoux S. Relation between infant feeding and infections during the first six months of life. *J Pediatrics*. 1995; **126**: 191–7.

22 Lopez-Alarcon M, Villalpando S, Fajardo A. Breastfeeding lowers the frequency and duration of acute respiratory infection and diarrhea in infants under six months of age. *J Nutr Educ*. 1997; **127**: 436–43.

23 Bachrach VR, Schwarz E, Bachrach LR. Breastfeeding and the risk of hospitalisation for respiratory disease in infancy: a meta-analysis. *Arch Pediatr Adolesc Med*. 2003; **157**: 237–43.

24 Oddy WH, Sly PD, de Klerk NH *et al*. Breastfeeding and respiratory morbidity in infancy: a birth cohort study. *Arch Dis Child*. 2003; **88**: 224–8.

25 Wilson A, Forsyth SA, Greene SA *et al.*, op. cit.

26 Saarinen UM. Prolonged breastfeeding as prophylaxis for recurrent otitis media. *Acta Paediatr Scand*. 1982; **71**: 567–71.

27 Duncan B, Ey J, Holberg CJ *et al*. Exclusive breastfeeding for at least four months protects against otitis media. *Pediatrics*. 1993; **91**: 867–72.

28 Paradise JL, Elster BA, Tan L. Evidence in infants with cleft palate that breast milk protects against otitis media. *Pediatrics*. 1994; **94**: 853–60.

29 Aniansson G, Alm B, Andersson B *et al*. A prospective cohort study on breastfeeding and otitis media in Swedish infants. *Pediatr Infect Dis J*. 1994; **13**: 183–8.

30 Pisacane A, Graziano L, Zona G. Breastfeeding and urinary tract infection. *Lancet*. 1990; **336**: 50.

31 Marild S, Hansson S, Jodal U *et al*. Protective effect of breastfeeding against urinary tract infection. *Acta Paediatr Scand*. 2004; **93**: 164–8.

32 Gdalevich M, Mimouni D, Mimouni M. Breastfeeding and the risk of bronchial asthma in childhood: a systematic review with meta-analysis of prospective studies. *J Pediatr*. 2001; **139**: 261–6.

33 Mayer E, Hamman R, Gay P *et al*. Reduced risk of IDDM among breastfed children: the Colorado IDDM Registry. *Diabetes Care*. 1988; **37**: 1625–32.

34 Gerstein HC. Cow's milk exposure and type I diabetes mellitus. A critical overview of the clinical literature. *Diabetes Care*. 1994; **17**: 13–19.

35 Arenz S, Ruckerl R, Koletzko B *et al*. Breastfeeding and childhood obesity – a systematic review. *Int J Obes Relat Metab Disord*. 2004; **28**: 1247–56.

36 Armstrong J, Reilly J, Child Health Information Team, op. cit.

37 von Kries R, Koletzko B, Sauerwald T *et al.*, op. cit.

38 Owen CG, Whincup PH, Odoki K *et al.*, op. cit.

39 Fewtrell MS. The long-term benefits of having been breastfed. *Curr Paediatr.* 2004; **14:** 97–103.

40 Wilson A, Forsyth SA, Greene SA *et al.*, op. cit.

41 Collaborative Group on Hormonal Factors in Breast Cancer. Breast cancer and breast-feeding: collaborative reanalysis of individual data from 47 epidemiological studies in 30 countries including 50 302 women with breast cancer and 97 973 women without the disease. *Lancet.* 2002; **360:** 187–95.

42 World Cancer Research Fund. *Diet and Cancer Report 2007.* www.dietandcancerreport. org (accessed 8 October 2009).

43 Dykes F. Return to breastfeeding: a global health priority. *Br J Midwifery.* 1997; **5:** 344–9.

44 Thapa S, Short R, Potts M. Breastfeeding, birth spacing and their effects on child survival. *Nature.* 1988; **335:** 679–82.

45 Ibid.

46 Dykes F, op. cit.

47 Meikle J. 'Myths' stop women breastfeeding. *The Guardian,* 6 May 2004, p. 6.

48 Perry A. Breasts – the cleavage between form and function. *Midwifery Matters.* 2001; **89:** 12–14.

49 Khella AK, Fhim HI, Issa AH *et al.* Lactational amenorrhea as a method of family planning in Egypt. *Contraception.* 2004; **69:** 317–22.

50 Weimer J, op. cit.

51 Shepherd CK, Kevin KG, Carter H. Examining the correspondence of breastfeeding and bottle-feeding couples' infant feeding attitudes. *J Adv Nurs.* 2000; **31:** 651–60.

52 Zimmerman DR, Guttman N. 'Breast is best': knowledge among low-income mothers is not enough. *J Hum Lact.* 2001; **17:** 14–19.

53 Colin WB, Scott JA. Breastfeeding: reasons for starting, reasons for stopping and problems along the way. *Breastfeed Rev.* 2002; **10:** 13–19.

54 Obermeyer CM, Castle S. Back to nature? Historical and cross-cultural perspectives on barriers to optimal breastfeeding. *Med Anthropol.* 1997; **17:** 39–63.

55 McDougall L. Damning report reveals abuse facing breastfeeding mothers. *Sunday Herald,* 9 May 2004.

56 Riordan J, Gill-Hopple K. Breastfeeding care in multicultural populations. *J Obstet Gynecol Neonatal Nurs.* 2001; **30:** 216–23.

57 Ibid.

58 Shepherd CK, Kevin KG, Carter H, op. cit.

59 Jackson KB. Women, men, breastfeeding and sexuality. *Br J Midwifery.* 2000; **8:** 83–6.

60 Thapa S, Short R, Potts M, op. cit.

61 Deacon C. Whose breasts are they anyway? *New Generation.* 1998; **17.**

62 Thapa S, Short R, Potts M, op. cit.

63 Deacon C, op. cit.

64 Renfrew MJ, Dyson L, Wallace L *et al. The Effectiveness of Public Health Interventions to Promote the Duration of Breastfeeding. Systematic review.* London: National Institute for Health and Clinical Excellence; 2005. www.nice.org.uk/page.aspx?o=511622 (accessed 5 October 2009).

65 McIntosh J. Barriers to breastfeeding: choice of feeding method in a sample of working-class primiparae. *Midwifery.* 1985; **1:** 213–24.

66 Gribble J. An alternative approach. *New Generation.* 1996; **15.**

67 Matthews K, Webber K, McKim E *et al.* Maternal infant-feeding decisions: reasons and influences. *Can J Nurs Res.* 1998; **30**: 177–98.

68 Colin WB, Scott JA, op. cit.

69 Bick DE, MacArthur C, Lancashire RJ. What influences the uptake and early cessation of breastfeeding? *Midwifery.* 1998; **14**: 242–7.

70 Wylie J, Verber I. Why women fail to breast-feed: a prospective study from booking to 28 days post-partum. *J Hum Nutr Dietetics.* 1994; **7**: 115–20.

71 Bick DE, MacArthur C, Lancashire RJ, op. cit.

72 Ford K, Labbok, M. Who is breast-feeding? Implications of associated social and biomedical variables for research on the consequences of method of infant feeding. *Am J Clin Nutr.* 1990; **52**: 451–6.

73 Wylie J, Verber I, op. cit.

74 Bick DE, MacArthur C, Lancashire RJ, op. cit.

75 Clements MS, Mitchell EA, Wright SP *et al.* Influences on breastfeeding in south-east England. *Acta Paediatr.* 1997; **86**: 51–6.

76 Wambach KA, Cole C. Breastfeeding and adolescents. *J Obstet Gynecol Neonatal Nurs.* 2000; **29**: 282–94.

77 Libbus K, Bush TA, Hockman NM. Breastfeeding beliefs of low-income primigravidae. *Int J Nurs Stud.* 1997; **34**: 114–50.

78 Brownell K, Hutton L, Hartman J *et al.* Barriers to breastfeeding among African American adolescent mothers. *Clin Pediatr.* 2002; **41**: 669–73.

79 Shaw RL, Wallace LM, Bansal M. Is breast best? Perceptions of infant feeding. *Community Practitioner.* 2003; **76**: 299–303.

80 Dykes F, Griffiths H. Societal influences upon initiation and continuation of breast-feeding. *Br J Midwifery.* 1998; **6**: 76–80.

81 Ibid.

82 Riordan J, Gill-Hopple K, op. cit.

83 Bandura A. Self-efficacy: toward a unifying theory of behavioural change. *Psychol Rev.* 1977; **84**: 191–215.

84 Blythe R, Creedy D, Dennis CL *et al.* Effect of maternal confidence on breast-feeding duration: an application of breast-feeding self-efficacy theory. *Birth.* 2002; **29**: 278–84.

85 Bandura A. Self-efficacy: toward a unifying theory of behavioural change, op. cit.

86 Bandura A. Self-efficacy mechanism in human agency. *Am Psychol.* 1982; **37**: 122–47.

87 Dennis CL, Faux S. Development and psychometric testing of the breastfeeding self-efficacy scale. *Res Nurs Health.* 1999; **22**: 399–409.

88 O'Campo P, Faden RR, Gielen AC *et al.* Prenatal factors associated with breastfeeding duration: recommendations for prenatal interventions. *Birth.* 1992; **19**: 195–201.

89 Buxton KE, Gielen AC, Faden RR *et al.* Women intending to breastfeed: predictors of early infant feeding experiences. *Am J Prev Med.* 1991; **7**: 101–6.

90 Dennis CL, Faux S, op. cit.

91 Bandura A. Self-efficacy: toward a unifying theory of behavioural change, op. cit.

92 Blythe R, Creedy D, Dennis CL *et al.*, op. cit.

93 Dennis CL, Faux S, op. cit.

94 Ibid.

95 Dennis CL. The breastfeeding self-efficacy scale: psychometric assessment of the short form. *J Obstet Gynecol Neonatal Nurs.* 2006; **32**: 734–44.

96 Zimmerman DR, Guttman N, op. cit.

97 Hoddinott P, Pill R. Qualitative study of decisions about infant feeding among women in east end of London. *BMJ.* 1999; **318:** 30–34.

98 Hill J. Breastfeeding and sexuality: societal conflicts and expectations. *Br J Midwifery.* 1997; **5:** 350–54.

99 Libbus K, Bush TA, Hockman NM, op. cit.

100 Rose VA, Warrington VO, Linder R *et al.* Factors influencing infant feeding method in an urban community. *J Natl Med Assoc.* 2004; **96:** 325–31.

101 Saunders-Goldson S, Edwards QT. Factors associated with breastfeeding intentions of African-American women at military health care facilities. *Mil Med.* 2004; **169:** 111–16.

102 Shepherd CK, Kevin KG, Carter H, op. cit.

103 Ineichen B, Pierce M, Lawrenson R. Teenage mothers as breastfeeders: attitudes and behaviour. *J Adolesc.* 1997; **20:** 505–9.

104 O'Connor ML. Black teenagers get less encouragement to nurse, and breastfeed less, than other young mothers. *Fam Plann Perspect.* 1999; **31:** 46–7.

105 Dennis C, Hodnett E, Gallop R *et al.* The effect of peer support on breastfeeding duration among primiparous women: a randomized controlled trial. *Can Med Assoc J.* 2002; **166:** 21–8.

106 Hoddinott P, Pill R, op. cit.

107 Lee E, Furedi F. *Mothers' Experience of, and Attitudes to, Using Infant Formula in the Early Months.* 2005. www.kent.ac.uk/sspssr/staff/academic/lee/infant-formula-full.pdf (accessed 8 October 2009).

108 Rossiter JC. The effect of a culture-specific education program to promote breastfeeding among Vietnamese women in Sydney. *Int J Nurs Stud.* 1994; **31:** 369–79.

109 Duffy EP, Percival P, Kershaw E. Positive effects of an antenatal group teaching session on postnatal nipple pain, nipple trauma and breastfeeding rates. *Midwifery.* 1997; **13:** 189–96.

110 Cooper PJ, Murray L, Stein A. Psychosocial factors associated with the early termination of breast-feeding. *J Psychosom Res.* 1993; **37:** 171–6.

111 Lawson K, Tulloch MI. Breastfeeding duration: prenatal intentions and postnatal practices. *J Adv Nurs.* 1995; **22:** 841–9.

112 Humphreys AS, Thompson NJ, Miner KR. Intention to breastfeed in low-income pregnant women: the role of social support and previous experience. *Birth.* 1998; **25:** 169–74.

113 Matthews K, Webber K, McKim E *et al.*, op. cit.

114 Avery M, Duckett L, Dodgson J *et al.* Factors associated with very early weaning among primiparas intending to breastfeed. *Matern Child Health J.* 1998; **2:** 167–79.

115 Dennis C, Hodnett E, Gallop R *et al.* The effect of peer support on breastfeeding duration among primiparous women: a randomized controlled trial, op. cit.

116 Dennis CL. Breastfeeding initiation and duration: a 1990–2000 literature review. *J Obstet Gynecol Neonatal Nurs.* 2002; **31:** 12–32.

117 Coles EC, Cotter S, Valman HB. Increasing prevalence of breastfeeding. *BMJ.* 1978; **2:** 1122.

118 Friel JK, Hudson NI, Banoub S *et al.* The effect of a promotion campaign on attitudes of adolescent females towards breastfeeding. *Can J Public Health.* 1989; **80:** 195–9.

119 Fairbank L, O'Meara S, Renfrew MJ *et al.* A systematic review to evaluate the effectiveness of interventions to promote the initiation of breastfeeding. *Health Technol Assess.* 2000; 4: 1–171.

120 Protheroe L, Dyson L, Renfrew M. *The Effectiveness of Public Health Interventions to Promote the Initiation of Breastfeeding.* Evidence Briefing. London: Health Development Agency; 2003.

121 Fairbank L, O'Meara S, Renfrew MJ, *et al.*, op. cit.

122 Renfrew MJ, Dyson L, Wallace L *et al.*, op. cit.

123 Ibid.

124 Tedstone A, Dunce N, Aviles M *et al. Effectiveness of Interventions to Promote Healthy Feeding of Infants Under One Year of Age: review.* London: Health Education Authority; 1998. www.nice.org.uk/page.aspx?o=501963 (accessed 5 October 2009).

125 Fairbank L, O'Meara S, Renfrew MJ *et al.*, op. cit.

126 Protheroe L, Dyson L, Renfrew M, op. cit.

127 Renfrew MJ, Dyson L, Wallace L *et al.*, op. cit.

128 Dyson L, Renfrew MJ, McFadden A *et al. Promotion of Breastfeeding Initiation and Duration. Evidence into practice briefing.* London: National Institute for Health and Clinical Excellence; 2006.

129 Renfrew MJ, Dyson L, McFadden A *et al. Effective Action Briefing on the Initiation and Duration of Breastfeeding. Technical report.* London: National Institute for Health and Clinical Excellence; 2005.

Initiating breastfeeding: a time for change – listening to the experiences of mothers

One night my baby was unsettled so they took him away. I felt so sad lying in bed not knowing if he was crying for me, if it was me he wanted. I think that was the only bad experience I had in hospital. It's all so much easier for them to just take them away for a while.[1]

INTRODUCTION

So far we have established that the 1990s witnessed a turning point in globally led initiatives to protect, promote and support breastfeeding, and saw hospitals in some countries changing previously 'poor' practices.[2,3] Despite some controversy surrounding advice and support from professionals, the evidence suggests that professional help and advice in the initiation and maintenance of breastfeeding are also critical.[4-6] The importance of professional support generally for promotion, initiation and maintenance of breastfeeding has already been emphasised in Chapter 2.

There is an increased awareness not only of the effect of breastfeeding on the long-term health outcomes for the mother and child, but also of the challenges to successful breastfeeding and recognition of the complexity of choosing to breastfeed. Breastfeeding rates remain relatively low in the UK, the experiences of women remain mixed, and the lack of knowledge and skills of professionals, and poor hospital practices, are still of concern.[7-10] This chapter builds on the framework of the UNICEF/WHO Ten Steps to Successful Breastfeeding and the Seven Point Plan[11,12] to explore further the claim that the key to breastfeeding success is promotion and effective initiation.[13]

This chapter will focus on issues relating to initiation, including the physiological processes and changes for mother and baby related to the establishment of breastfeeding. Social, economic and psychological factors are also considered, as well as the potential emotional impact on the mother of starting to breastfeed. Throughout this chapter there are references to the Baby-Friendly practice standards, as reminders of the relevance of specific topics to these international standards.

INITIATION: THE TEN STEPS AND THE SEVEN POINT PLAN

The UNICEF/WHO Ten Steps to Successful Breastfeeding and Seven Point Plan are considered to be the key documents that provide health professionals with a foundation for best practice in the initiation and continuation of breastfeeding.[14,15] The experiences of women and breastfeeding outcomes were improved when these standards were implemented.[16] However, implementation of the standards has been relatively slow, and adoption of good practice varies from one country to another. It is clear that despite the gains made in the 1990s, the challenge of relatively low breastfeeding rates remains, and a great deal of work needs to be undertaken so that breastfeeding becomes the norm rather than the exception. National surveys in the UK are undertaken every five years, commissioned by the Department of Health. The decline in breastfeeding from birth until nine months remains evident, and breastfeeding mothers who deliver at full term encounter many breastfeeding problems during the first week of lactation.[17]

In the UK, the National Institute for Health and Clinical Excellence (NICE) provides an example of building on the successes of the past. The NICE postnatal guidelines recommend that providers of healthcare in both hospitals and community settings should put into practice a programme that actively supports breastfeeding, with the Baby-Friendly Initiative (BFI) used as the minimum standard.[18]

More recently, a review of the Seven Point Plan in the UK has been completed following an extensive national consultation. This critical review recognises the importance of adopting a multifaceted approach in the wider community when supporting women to continue to breastfeed in the community. Baby-Friendly accreditation is an important aspect of this, and information about the stages of assessment for Baby-Friendly accreditation in community settings can be found on the BFI website (www.babyfriendly.org.uk/page.asp?page=71).

UNDERSTANDING THE INITIATION OF BREASTFEEDING

Maternal and infant reflexes

There are a number of maternal and infant reflexes which work in physiological partnership to initiate breastfeeding and ensure its continuance.[19] Three complementary reflexes occur when the infant feeds, namely the physiological responses of rooting, sucking and swallowing. Each reflex has a specific function, but they work in harmony.

➤ The rooting reflex programmes the infant to search for the nipple.
➤ The sucking reflex coordinates a rhythmic jaw action creating negative pressure and a peristaltic action of the tongue.
➤ The swallowing reflex ensures that the milk is regularly removed from the mouth to avoid choking and aspiration.

The two maternal reflexes involved in lactation are the milk production reflex and the milk ejection reflex. Both involve the production of hormones – prolactin for milk production, and oxytocin for milk ejection. Stimulation by the infant of nerve endings in the nipple/areolar complex sends impulses through afferent neural-reflex pathways to the hypothalamus. This stimulates a response action and results in the secretion of prolactin from the anterior pituitary gland and oxytocin from the posterior pituitary gland.

Prolactin is a key lactogenic hormone, and it stimulates initial alveolar production of milk. Prolactin receptor sites in the acini cells of the alveoli need to be primed by the hormone prolactin during the first few days of lactation. If the pituitary gland produces insufficient prolactin to be released into the bloodstream, these sites shut down and cannot be reopened. The importance of early and frequent feeding is therefore crucial to the establishment of lactation. Hospital practices such as delayed feeding, separation of mother and infants, and the use of teats and dummies have all played a significant role in poor milk production.

Oxytocin contracts the myo-epithelial cells, forcing the milk from the ducts.[20] The milk ejection reflex is very powerful, as it responds to visual, olfactory and auditory stimulation. It can be triggered in some mothers by physical closeness to their baby or simply by thinking about the infant. The force of the contraction of the alveoli can also be strong and painful. Mothers may feel the let-down as a warm tingling sensation in the breast which may be accompanied by an itchy feeling. Where milk removal is ineffective, a suppressor peptide present locally in the breast tissue as the feedback inhibitor of lactation (FIL) will increase and inhibit milk production.[21]

Induced lactation

In developing countries there is a long history of mothers inducing lactation.[22,23] This may be a relevant issue for adoptive mothers who have not experienced pregnancy but who want to bond with their baby through breastfeeding. With the correct information, support and advice, lactation can be initiated within a matter of weeks. In a study of six Nigerian women where the mother of the infant had died, lactation was induced within 3 to 4 weeks.[24] In a Papua New Guinea study, a combination of milk-stimulating drugs and baby-led feeding resulted in a full milk supply in 88% of cases.[25]

Breastfeeding more than one infant

As milk production is determined by supply and demand, stimulation by two infants produces sufficient milk for both babies. Therefore the breastfeeding of twins should not present a physiological problem with milk supply in respect of demand.[26] This is also the case in situations where the mother may be malnourished or not have access to a healthy diet.[27,28] The challenge for the mother is coping with the demands of two or more babies. This may be an overwhelming experience for the mother, especially immediately after the birth and when initiating breastfeeding.

Each situation has its own unique set of variables associated with the physical and psychological make-up of the mother and babies, and the social and cultural context in which the breastfeeding is taking place. The mother's individual needs are particularly important with respect to physiological factors, such as stamina and tiredness levels, and psychological factors, such as self-efficacy, previous experience, availability of experienced professional support and having a social support system in place. When the mother feels confident about attachment and the infants have 'learned' correct attachment, the mother should be offered support to feed the babies simultaneously.[29] This provides the mother with a choice of approach to feeding, which is less time-consuming and may be of help when she is feeling tired.

Many mothers of twins find that the demands of both infants coincide. Feeding simultaneously avoids a situation where the mother becomes anxious because one baby is left to cry while the other is being fed.[30] Mothers may thus gain physical and psychological benefits from feeding in tandem. Feeding simultaneously is a skill that needs to be learned. Mothers therefore require time, support and the opportunity to gain dexterity and to develop confidence and patience. Reassurance from the professional and relevant others is a necessary and important aspect of the learning process, and will have long-term benefits.

Physiological preparation for breastfeeding

Lactogenesis is the production of milk by the mammary glands. The point at which the developing breasts have the capacity to synthesise milk constituents and secrete milk is referred to as lactogenesis 1. Lactogenesis II occurs when the milk volume has increased over a period of 24–48 hours. This natural preparation process is so effective that lactation could take place even if the pregnancy discontinued at 16 weeks.[31] After delivery, the placental inhibition of milk synthesis no longer occurs, and the progesterone levels in the blood decrease.

Colostrum is a high-density, low-volume, sticky, yellowish fluid, which fills the alveolar cells in the breast during the last trimester of pregnancy and is available immediately before the delivery and for the first few days following the delivery. The amounts of colostrum secreted vary widely from one individual to another, ranging from 10 to 100 ml/day, with a mean of 30 ml/day.[32] The evolution of colostrum into mature milk is highly dependent on individual circumstances, and can occur between 3 and 14 days after delivery.

Colostrum contains less lactose, fat and water-soluble vitamins than mature milk, but more protein and fat-soluble vitamins (E, A and K), and more of the minerals zinc and sodium. The soluble components include immunoglobulins (IgA, IgM and IgG), lysozymes, enzymes, lactoferrin, the bifidus factor and immunoregulatory substances. The anti-infective agents in colostrum have both soluble and cellular components.[33] The cellular components include macrophages, lymphocytes, neutrophil granulocytes and epithelial cells. Colostrum therefore contains protective factors and is a reliable and abundant source of immunoglobulins.

The immunoglobulins that are found in colostrum provide a degree of protection to the infant, especially in organs such as the lungs and the gastrointestinal tract. For example, the immunoglobulins coat the lining of the infant's gut, preventing the adherence of bacterial, viral, parasitic and other pathogens. In addition, the bifidus factor in colostrum is a nitrogen-containing carbohydrate, which promotes intestinal colonisation with lactobacilli in the presence of lactose. This results in a low pH in the intestinal lumen, which inhibits the growth of *E. coli*, Gram-negative bacteria and fungi.

The innate ability of the newborn

The human newborn has an innate ability to find and attach at the breast and feed. Self-attachment depends partly on smell. Where a mother has unwashed nipples her newborn infant is four times more likely to attach at the breast than in the case of a mother with washed nipples.[34] Infants will also crawl towards the smell of an object that has been in contact with the breast, such as a breast pad.[35] The newborn infant also has the ability to recognise their own mother's face,[36] responds better to their own mother's face,[37] and demonstrates in the absence of maternal body contact a separation distress call.[38] There is therefore a requirement that this physiological ability, which is unique to mammals, should be recognised and afforded a degree of priority over routine hospital practices. The task-orientated delivery ward environment at the time of birth can take priority over skin-to-skin contact and ensuring that successful first feeds take place, hence the importance of this standard within the Ten Steps to Successful Breastfeeding:

> Help mothers to initiate breastfeeding soon after birth.
>
> (Baby-Friendly practice standard)

Skin-to-skin contact

A Cochrane literature review of 17 studies provides evidence that skin-to-skin contact has a positive impact on long-term breastfeeding, with no negative effects identified.[39] Skin-to-skin contact should therefore be encouraged as early as possible to help with successful initiation and to support continuation. There is evidence that this early contact during the first feed, in the delivery room, is important because it has a positive effect on breastfeeding outcome.[40,41] Skin contact has both physical and psychological benefits, and should continue uninterrupted for at least half an hour, particularly after separation has occurred.[42,43] An added advantage of skin contact for ill or premature infants is that it is more likely to maintain body temperature, regulate breathing and heart rate, improve oxygen saturation and encourage breastfeeding.[44–46]

Mothers who do not wish or are unable to breastfeed will benefit physiologically and physically from skin-to skin-contact.[47,48] Practices in hospital or the community should ensure that mothers are supported and encouraged to have as much close skin-to-skin contact as possible, as soon as possible after delivery and thereafter. Certain factors may reduce the potential for skin-to-skin contact. For example, a number of studies have found that the administration of pethidine during labour is associated with disorganised sucking and shorter breastfeeding duration.[49–51] Health professionals should be alerted to the fact that mothers who have been given pethidine may require additional support to achieve skin-to-skin contact and to initiate breastfeeding.[52]

Practice expert

The evidence on breastfeeding and skin-to-skin contact and bonding is clear, and should be reinforced through community and hospital policies during antenatal and postnatal care. Fundamental to practices that aim to promote, protect and support breastfeeding is the use of strategies that preserve and nurture the relationship between mother and child, from the moment of birth.

Vignette: Mismatch of policy and practice – the mother's perspective

'I know that it's mostly policy to hand the baby to the mothers straight away and try and get them to feed as soon as possible, and I did find it quite odd that didn't happen.'

Reflect

What policies and practices should be in place to avoid a repetition of the situation described in the above vignette, and to ensure that mothers are enabled to challenge practices that are not compatible with supporting breastfeeding, rather than being obstructed from doing so?

Show mothers how to breastfeed and how to maintain lactation even if they are separated from their babies.

(Baby-Friendly practice standard)

Breastfeeding is a learned process

Breastfeeding is not necessarily an instinctive behaviour in all women. Woolridge suggests that correct attachment of the baby to the breast is a skill which is acquired by observation and practice.[53] In some developing countries, breastfeeding is more of a social event than in Western societies, and young women have had the opportunity to learn from experienced women in their social circle. In other countries, this experience has been lost through the introduction of formula feeding. As we established in Chapter 2, in societies where there are few or no opportunities to embody knowledge through exposure and subsequent attitude formation, and where breastfeeding is no longer the norm, mothers may not have the advantage of learning how to breastfeed through observation.

There is therefore a strong element of learning involved in initiation of breastfeeding. In developed countries it has been found that mothers who have attended breastfeeding workshops, and who have had access to information about breastfeeding prior to delivery, are more confident about their ability to breastfeed.[54] According to Renfrew *et al*, it is also crucial that all breastfeeding mothers have the full support of an experienced health professional in the early stages of breastfeeding, that the professional should regard each mother-and-baby relationship as unique and individualised, and that assessment, support and advice should be managed on this principle.[55]

Knowledge of normal infant behaviour, infant cues, positioning and attachment, and the ability to problem solve and troubleshoot through the presenting challenges and difficulties, are essential. Mothers need this expert support in order to avoid problems and ensure breastfeeding success. Most mothers will require assistance and reassurance over several feeds, and possibly over several days and at particular times. Continuity of information giving is also a vital part of initiating and maintaining the learning process, and contributes to subsequent success and confidence.

Practice expert

Managers and clinicians have a joint responsibility to ensure that despite the busy environment of a hospital department, the individual needs of a breastfeeding mother are met, especially a mother who is initiating breastfeeding for the first time.

Vignette: Protecting and supporting women who are breastfeeding

'I mean I do appreciate that they are busy on the wards, but even if they were to take the time out when you are ready to feed, you know, you have to buzz for them and if somebody was available to come around and say right, well, you show us the way you put them on and we will then show you where you are going right or not, and this is the way you should be doing it you know, but I didn't feel that was the way they did it, it was just more get them on and that's it, so I was buzzing them all of the time, and he wouldn't go on because it was like I can't get him on, but they were just coming around and putting him on and that was it and then they were away.'

Reflect

How can professionals balance the need to 'get the work done' with the individual needs of the mother who is breastfeeding?

Enabling good positioning and attachment

It is normal for a mother's breasts to feel tender after the first day of breastfeeding, because the baby's first sucks stretch the areola tissue back into the mouth. Nipple tenderness at the beginning of feeding is normal in the first two to three days of breastfeeding. This usually lessens when the milk lets down, and it should disappear completely within a few days. Soreness that is intense or that occurs later indicates the need to assess feeding position and attachment. A mother who learns to position her baby well and attach him or her correctly can expect little or no nipple tenderness. In most cases, sore cracked nipples or bleeding nipples can be alleviated by adjusting the position.

How well the mother and baby are positioned in relation to each other will dictate how well the baby attaches to the breast for the first feed, and will influence the success of breastfeeding initiation. The following key principles can be used as guidance.

➤ Ensure that the mother is comfortable, whether she is sitting up or lying down, and provide support for her back and feet if required. Advise and reassure her that breasts vary in shape and size. The position of the nipple will also vary. It is therefore important to advise her not to lift the breast to the baby, but to take the baby to the position where the nipple naturally sits.

➤ Encourage the mother to hold her baby close to her body, supporting the baby's whole body in a straight line, avoiding the baby twisting their neck and shoulders. The baby should be facing the breast, with their nose opposite the nipple.

➤ Teach the mother to recognise early feeding cues, such as licking the lips, sticking out the tongue, rooting, finger sucking, looking intently, and eagerness to feed. Crying is usually the last cue. Encourage the mother to talk to her baby, and to look at and encourage the baby. Advise her to stimulate the gape reflex and wait for a wide open mouth, then bring the baby quickly to the breast leading with the chin, aiming her nipple at the roof of her baby's mouth, with the bottom lip well away from the base of the nipple. This essentially means that the baby will lead with the chin.

➤ The feed will begin with rapid sucks, which will change to deeper more rhythmic sucks with swallows. The baby will be calm and stay on the breast throughout the whole feed.

➤ During the feed the cheeks will appear full and rounded, and the chin will indent the breast. The mouth will look wide open and the lower lip may be turned outwards, although it is not always possible to see this. Depending on the size of the mother's areola, there will be more visible at the top than below.

➤ At the end of the feed the baby will release the breast and will look satisfied and sleepy. The nipple will be the same shape as the beginning of the feed.

There are various assessment tools to enable helpers to check the positioning and attachment, but the above principles are generally used as a common foundation.

Practice expert

The manner in which the healthcare professional approaches the attachment of the baby to the breast in preparation for feeding, and the accuracy of a feeding assessment, both contribute substantially to the mother's experience of breastfeeding. Professionals must be aware of the 'push and pull' mechanisms that exist in day-to-day practice, such as the need to commit time to supporting the mother to attach the infant to the breast, and to balance this against the pressure to complete certain tasks within a given time period. The latter can lead to the tendency to apply a 'one size fits all' approach in practice, with a loss of sensitivity to the individual needs of women who are trying to establish breastfeeding.

Vignette: The right support at the right time in the right manner

'I felt quite as if I was being invaded. They just grabbed it, opened the baby's mouth, shoving my nipple in, and it was like head on and everything just seemed to be getting pushed and pulled and then it was like that's it, the baby is on, so I am away.'

'The midwives really were helping, they tried everything – they were squeezing my breasts, I felt like a cow being milked.'

'We stayed in hospital for five days, and I think two or three times we had help from a breastfeeding specialist. She came round and when she was helping, he latched on fine, but the other times with the midwives there it was humiliating.'

'They [the midwives] would just come and man-handle you, like shoving your nipple in his mouth. I think at one point I had two midwives like basically trying to get my baby to feed, and I was just lying there feeling like a complete weed. I looked at them and thought "I'm not needed here at all." They weren't talking to me and they weren't involving me in it. It was awful.'

Reflect

The skill, expertise and competence required by the professional to support breastfeeding cannot be over-emphasised. Enabling mothers to position and attach their baby is fundamental to breastfeeding success. In a review of the qualitative literature, many mothers described experiencing a physically intrusive, distressing and embarrassing 'hands-on' approach. Mothers also reported experiencing difficulty in achieving this skill themselves when it had been done for them by the health professional.[56] Observe and reflect on how sensitive, empathetic and caring the facilitation of attachment is in local practice. How effective is the communication between professional(s) and the mother, particularly in relation to observation of the mother's non-verbal cues?

Tongue tie

Infants with a short frenulum may experience difficulty with attachment and with staying attached. The infant may also be fretful and unable to extend the tongue adequately from the mouth. In cases where this is interfering with good attachment, a frenectomy will support continuation with breastfeeding,[57-59] and in the UK a national referral system is in place to support this. If the infant appears to have a short frenulum and this is affecting breastfeeding, healthcare professionals can make a referral. More information about the UK referral system is available on the UK UNICEF Baby-Friendly website (www.babyfriendly.org. uk/page.asp?page=153).

In the UK, training for healthcare professionals to enable them to perform this procedure is also available.

Flat or inverted nipples

If the mother has flat or inverted nipples, attachment may be more challenging. However, Hoffman exercises to stretch inverted nipples and any other types of preparation are not recommended during pregnancy.[60] Women will need to be given a careful explanation of the physiology so that they understand about the need to express breast milk, if the attachment is initially unsuccessful. It will take time and patience to assist and encourage the mother to continue with her efforts to breastfeed. The mother and baby will both require time. Milk expression should be implemented to ensure effective breast stimulation and avoid an increase in FIL. Skin-to-skin contact and frequent offers to breastfeed are also necessary to facilitate and support the development of skills in attachment. Breast shells, breast pumps and other aids can be used prior to feeds, to encourage the nipple to protrude. The situation needs to be managed with patience by an experienced professional, over a period of time, during the postnatal period.

Baby-led feeding.

(Baby-Friendly practice standard)

The more often a baby feeds at the breast, the more breast milk will be produced for the next feed. This unique physiological and hormonal relationship is based on a supply-and-demand partnership. The volume of milk that is produced depends on how well the infant attaches to the breast and how efficient their sucking is in removing milk from the breast. This partnership is unique to each mother and baby. Mothers who breastfeed on demand have a large volume of milk by 24–48 hours after birth, but with the firstborn infant it can take a few days longer to establish the volume of milk.

This process is often described as milk 'coming in', and it marks the change from endocrine control of lactation to autocrine control. It is associated with a sensation of fullness and increased warmth in the breasts. The increasing fullness is due to a combination of inefficient milk removal and increased blood flow. Problems associated with fullness occur when lymphatic oedema builds up in the breast and limits the outflow of milk. If allowed to continue, this situation will eventually cause an accumulation of suppressor peptides or FIL, which are responsible for a reduction in milk supply.

Practice expert

Hormonal stimulation and future milk production are crucial. However, it is important to be alert to possible literal interpretation, where a mother may leave a newborn infant without attempting to rouse them for feeding for several hours. This is equally hazardous to milk production. In some situations, as a result of allowing baby-led feeding, there have been reports of periods of up to 12 hours without feeding or expressing milk from the breast. This will have a direct impact on milk production.

Vignette: Restricted feeding and consequent milk supply

'They said she is not getting enough and to wake her, but I just felt that if they wanted food they would wake up for it. I thought if they are content to sleep they are obviously not hungry. After a feed she was content to go back to sleep for 4 to 6 hours, so she was obviously getting what she needed. I don't produce a lot of milk, for whatever reason, and the fact that they are big babies may have something to do with it.'

Reflect

This mother of three introduced formula milk to all of her children by 3 weeks of age, where their growth was a cause for concern. The advice given, although appropriate in terms of stimulating milk production, did not appear to be understood in terms of real consequences to her milk supply.

It is important to adopt an approach which ensures that prolactin stimulation and milk production continue uninterrupted. Supplements should therefore be avoided, and the mother should be encouraged to offer the baby regular feeds in the early days following the birth, and should be supported in developing awareness and learning to respond to feeding cues from the baby. Decisions to change from exclusive breastfeeding should not be taken lightly, and should be preceded by a detailed and expert assessment of infant attachment and positioning. Careful and considered assessment of such a situation is therefore a key area in breastfeeding practice. The most important component is to ensure full understanding by the mother about the management and advice provided.

> Give newborn infants no food or drink other than breast milk, unless medically indicated.
>
> (Baby-Friendly practice standard)

It has been known for over a decade that when breastfeeding is effective, water or formula supplements are not required.[61] Supplementation may complicate breastfeeding and undermine self-efficacy at a time when the mother may be physically and psychologically vulnerable. In a study by Wylie and Verber, insufficient milk was the commonest reason cited by mothers for stopping breastfeeding.[62] These findings were supported almost a decade later by the results of the Infant Feeding Survey, which identified that supplementing breast-feeding with bottles of formula showed the strongest association with early cessation of breastfeeding.[63]

Practice expert

The delivery of healthcare is based not on the concept of collective responsibility, but on individual accountability. Each professional therefore has sole responsibility for ensuring that their practice is up to date and increasingly evidence based. In the following vignette the evidence for not supplementing, which has been consistent and continuous since the early 1990s and remains so in the current evidence, was ignored.

Vignette: The research is clear – do not supplement

'I wanted to breastfeed and they wanted to give him a bottle of milk, but I was scared that would make him not want to breastfeed, but they were kind of insisting on this.'

'I gave her formula as they said it would be a treat for her and so she could sleep.'

'They wanted to give him formula, but I was scared it would put him off breastfeeding.'

'I was left to get on with it as she was my second baby. She was always underweight, and I was told by the paediatrician to give formula. I tried all the ways to increase my supply, but she always had one bottle a day, which made me sad.'

Reflect

In the above vignette the instincts of the women were more accurate and correct than the practice of the professionals. Consider the importance of having current knowledge of breastfeeding policy. Consider also how to ensure that practice and competence are kept up to date. Locally, how much practice is evidence based? What are the mechanisms for ensuring that knowledge of current research in this area is kept up to date?

Cultural reasons for introducing supplements

In some cultures, pre-lacteal feeds (e.g. herbal teas, ghee or banana) are given for ritual purposes.[64] This is done in the belief that colostrum is harmful, and the aim of these supplements is therefore to clean the infant's gut. In some societies the first breastfeed may be delayed for days and colostrum discarded.[65] However, the evidence suggests that infants who receive pre-lacteal formula feeds are less likely to be fully breastfeeding at 6 weeks, and there is a direct relationship between the number of pre-lacteal feeds received and the likelihood of not breastfeeding.[66]

Medical reasons for introducing supplements

There are a number of acceptable medical reasons for providing supplementary feeds to a newborn infant. The reasons are varied and may be transient, so every effort must be made to encourage and support the developing milk supply until breastfeeding is possible. An important principle of practice is that the use of supplements without a medical indication is associated with earlier cessation of breastfeeding.[67-70] A further principle of practice is that if an infant is allowed to demand feed, has unrestricted feeding frequency and duration, and is correctly attached at the breast, milk production should be sustained adequately throughout lactation. If the continuity of lactation is interrupted, reasonable steps need to be taken to maintain lactation. The following medical reasons may cause lactation to be interrupted:

➤ maternal medication contraindicated during breastfeeding
➤ severe intrauterine growth retardation
➤ severe hypoglycaemia, which may result in intrauterine growth restriction (IUGR) due to hyperinsulinaemia
➤ inborn errors of metabolism (e.g. phenylketonuria, galactosaemia or maple syrup urine disease)
➤ acute neonatal dehydration or hypernatraemia
➤ maternal illness (e.g. psychosis, eclampsia or shock).

Where supplementation is necessary and medically indicated, avoiding the use of teats to administer the supplement is recommended. The practice of switching between breast and bottle feeds with teats can cause nipple confusion in the baby, due to the different suck techniques, and may lead to breast refusal.[71]

Mothers may request that formula is given to their infant even when these medical conditions are absent. Careful discussion should then take place with the mother to ensure that she makes a fully informed choice. In such instances professionals can use the information in the Ten Steps and the Seven Point Plan to guide informed decision making. Another consideration is that early exposure to cow's milk may put infants who are genetically susceptible at risk of developing allergic conditions such as asthma and eczema.[72-74]

An empathetic understanding and unhurried approach can help when a mother is at the point of requesting formula milk. This is often related to exhaustion, sore nipples, or a difficult and fretful infant who remains unsettled after frequent feeding. Spending time listening and responding to the mother's concerns is an integral part of responsive management. Inclusion of the following strategies can provide the all-important encouragement to continue with breastfeeding, and can also help to sustain milk supply during a period of medically indicated supplementation:

➤ support with skin-to-skin contact
➤ help with understanding the behaviour of the baby when there is skin-to-skin contact
➤ help with positioning and attachment, and remaining with the mother for the full feed, describing what is happening
➤ help with expressing breast milk
➤ help with understanding feeding cues to enable baby-led feeding
➤ help with avoiding the use of teats and dummies for giving expressed breast milk.

The WHO's International Code of Marketing of Breast-Milk Substitutes supports informed choice for mothers and highlights the importance of providing accurate information.[75] The decision by a mother to give her baby supplementary feeds should therefore be supported by documented evidence of discussions about practices to support breastfeeding as outlined above, and the known adverse effects of supplementation.

Practise rooming in.

(Baby-Friendly practice standard)

'Rooming in' refers to a situation where the baby remains with the mother following the birth. For over a generation, rooming in has been a topic of concern and debate. Despite clear evidence of the value of rooming in to the mother, her partner and the baby, professionals have been slow to adopt the rooming in practice.[76,77] The reasons for this may be linked to traditional professional and personal attitudes towards care during childbirth. Decisions by organisations to provide rooming in accommodation may also be influenced by additional economic and political factors.

Practice expert
The separation of mother and baby is a last resort, and should only occur under exceptional circumstances (e.g. if the baby requires specialist treatment). Even then, all efforts should be concentrated on reducing the separation as much as possible. Women need to be encouraged to ask questions and, where necessary, to challenge practices that they feel are not appropriate or about which they are unhappy.

Vignette: Separation is not the answer

'One night my baby was unsettled, so they took him away. I felt so sad lying in bed not knowing if he was crying for me, if it was me he wanted. I think that was the only bad experience I had in hospital. It's all so much easier for them to just take them away for a while. I think because he was feeding constantly they gave the reason that he was smelling the milk off me and that's what he wants all the time, and that they would take him away for half an hour and bring him back and try and settle him. But they never brought him back.'

Reflect

It was established earlier that listening to women and providing a safe environment that encourages them to 'speak up' is a fundamental principle of supporting breastfeeding. Does this working principle extend into hospital practices?

Rooming in policy and practice

Avoiding the separation of mother and baby supports breastfeeding practice, especially during the crucial phase of initiating breastfeeding. Rooming in therefore has a positive effect on lactation, as it allows greater frequency of feeding and has been associated with faster weight gain[78] and higher rates of exclusive breastfeeding, which have a longer duration.[79] A policy of 24-hour rooming in can reduce the problem of separation of mothers from their babies at night, which is a factor known to contribute to the early introduction of formula feeds.[80] It also enables the traditional practice of offering a good night's sleep following labour to be challenged using evidence to support the fact that the quality and quantity of sleep that women achieve when separation occurs is found to be poor, due to anxieties about their infant's welfare during the separation.[81]

Separation of mother from an ill or preterm infant

Bennett and Slade have highlighted the acute psychological distress experienced by mothers when their baby is unwell at the time of or shortly after the birth, and many mothers reported feeling guilt, anxiety, fear and helplessness.[82] The family that is caught up in this situation has to cope with and overcome a series of emotional hurdles before contemplating the role of parent. Giving women the knowledge that they require to make informed decisions about their infant's care, including the initiation of breastfeeding, empowers them to make choices and helps to restore their self-confidence and sense of self-worth.[83–86] Establishing breastfeeding in a way that facilitates the continuation and success of breastfeeding will depend on how well individual situations are managed.

If an infant needs to be admitted to hospital or to a specialist preterm infant unit, the importance of initiating breastfeeding may be overlooked, as understandably the overriding objective is the well-being of the baby or babies. Providing the mother with information on expressing milk and initiating breastfeeding is particularly important during the initial hours and days follow-ing the delivery. Ideally, expression of breast milk should take place within 6 hours of delivery.

Coping with the stress of an ill or preterm baby has additional consequences for the emotional well-being of the family.[87] Despite this, there is an increas-ing awareness that in the presence of illness or prematurity, women remain motivated to provide breast milk for their babies.[88] Furthermore, separation of the baby from the mother, on the grounds of allowing the mother rest and opportunity to sleep, has been shown not to result in a significant difference in the amount or quality of the mother's sleep, compared with leaving the mother and baby together.[89]

Preterm infants benefit greatly from being breastfed, as the breast milk con-tains significantly higher concentrations of protein and minerals than full-term human milk, making it more suitable for the premature infant.[90] Initiating breastfeeding in a preterm baby also has a beneficial effect on neurodevelop-ment.[91] Even when breast milk needs to be supplemented, promotion, support and initiation of breastfeeding for the premature infant lead to physical and psychological benefits for the baby and the mother.[92] Expression of breast milk may provide comfort to the mother. Therefore reassurance, advice and support on expressing breast milk must be continuous, and should be initiated as soon as possible after the birth of the baby.[93] It is advised that professional help should be available on the first day, and expression performed six to eight times in 24 hours, with at least one night-time expression.[94]

The research evidence suggests that if the infant's life is at risk, the mother may feel compromised with regard to her emotions towards her baby, and it may be that only when she feels sure her baby will survive does she find it easier to relax and allow her feelings for the baby to develop.[95] This situation may have a direct impact on the woman's decision to breastfeed, but helping her to keep her options open is particularly important at any time. As milk production is emotionally and hormonally driven, the milk supply will fluctuate according to the baby's condition and that of the mother. Continuous reassurance is essential.

> Give no artificial teats or dummies to breastfeeding infants.
>
> (Baby-Friendly practice standard)

The use of artificial teats and pacifiers is common practice in many Western socie-ties, and it presents a constant challenge to the establishment and continuation of breastfeeding.

The controversy about the use of artificial teats and pacifiers arises because of the mechanical difference in sucking technique, the problems stemming from this, and nipple confusion in the baby. The early introduction of a paci-fier (e.g. within 2 to 5 days of birth), compared with late introduction (at more than 4 weeks), has been found to shorten the duration of breastfeeding.[96,97] The use of a pacifier may be an indicator of difficulties in breastfeeding or reduced motivation to breastfeed.[98] Nipple confusion has been reported as a result of the introduction of pacifiers, and has been found to lead to breast refusal, resulting in a reduction in milk supply due to inappropriate or diminished sucking strength.[99-101]

Nipple shields are traditionally used in Western societies when a mother has flat or inverted nipples, large breasts and sore or cracked nipples, but the use of a nipple shield has been associated with a preference of the infant for the rubber nipple of the shield, resulting in refusal to attach to the breast.[102] Importantly, the use of nipple shields reduces milk production, triggering a downward spiral of events, with the baby surviving on milk that is leaking into the shield due to the milk ejection reflex, accompanied by inadequate emptying or stimulating of the breast.[103] Similarly, the practice of switching between breast and bottle feeds can cause nipple confusion in the baby due to the different sucking techniques involved, and may lead to breast refusal.[104] It should also be recognised that nipple shields may be used to protect breastfeeding, as demonstrated in the account below. It is advisable that where nipple shields are used there is a strategy for stopping their use.

There are reports that preterm infants can be offered alternative feeding methods, including cup feeding,[105] nasogastric tube feeding,[106] finger feeding[107] and paladai, a traditional Indian feeding device.[108] A Cochrane review found that supplementing breastfeeds by cup confers no breastfeeding benefit beyond discharge home, and delays discharge considerably.[109] However, the preterm infant benefits enormously from breastfeeding. Exclusive breastfeeding rates at discharge were significantly higher where cup feeding was used as an intervention during the hospital stay. Consideration of the factors that influence continuation in the community and ways to provide additional support for this population are recommended.

Practice expert
The evidence suggests that nipple confusion caused by the use of nipple shields or bottle teats can impede, delay or prevent the establishment of breastfeeding. The following vignette again highlights the importance of current knowledge and of basing professional practice on research evidence.

Vignette: Support in action
'He didn't latch on for about 3 weeks. I had to use nipple shields and had to express most of the milk and feed it to him through a bottle. I was so annoyed that it wasn't working. If it had happened more easily I don't know if I would have stuck to it. The first 3 weeks were so hard.'

Reflect

The persistence and determination demonstrated by this particular mother were evident. However, there is a strong indication that additional support is required when events are not straightforward. There is growing acceptance of attempts to utilise measures that may be beneficial at an individual level following assessment, but there is also an additional need to follow through the support in order to minimise the anxiety that is experienced in this situation.

Practice expert

This all-important individual assessment and support is beneficial to the mother–infant dyad, as is demonstrated in the following vignette by a mother who was faced with a combination of issues that had an impact on effective positioning and attachment.

Vignette: Support, tailored by individual assessment

'Instead of getting resentful and stubborn about what I was being told to do, I was getting resentful and stubborn about the fact that we couldn't do it right. I thought "We're going to do it, we're not going to give up until it actually happens", so we carried on and we're still breastfeeding.'

Reflect

Interestingly, this mother viewed herself and the baby as being in a partnership which was supported and reinforced by her support networks, professionals and the family unit. A crucial component was the planning and effective communication to enable joint decision making by both the healthcare professional supporting this mother to persevere, and the mother herself. Despite the difficulties that were encountered, the ultimate goal of establishing breastfeeding was achieved through a belief that eventually this would in fact be the outcome. For many similar breastfeeding challenges it is the invisible but all-important belief that is instilled in the mother which contributes to success.

Practice expert

A professional who has knowledge and skills with regard to attachment may forget how unfamiliar and threatening this aspect of breastfeeding can be for women, especially those who are breastfeeding for the first time, and those who have previously had a negative experience. To a greater or lesser extent, the majority of women experience the feelings that are expressed in the following vignette.

Vignette: Careful assessment with caring, consistent and continuous support

'When I first had C, it took a couple of days for us to get used to breastfeeding, and it was learning for both of us, and for me to calm down about it because you are obviously very nervous. He wasn't really feeding the first couple of days. He was 4 weeks early. A lot of the nurses at the hospital are all really helpful, but then all the different information is too much to take in and wasn't all the same thing. As a mum that got confusing, because you are anxious about the whole process anyway, and it is not that they were wrong, it was just that they didn't all say the same thing.'

'There was one particular nurse who came to help out and she was fantastic. She dealt with me all day, and she just stuck to what she said and didn't deviate from it. She wasn't mixing me up, and said this is what we are doing and you just have to stick to it. It was really good, and she helped a lot. When we came home I actually stayed in for an extra day because I wasn't happy breastfeeding and wasn't satisfied that I would be able to come home and do it myself. After the day with that lady everything was great, and I came home and felt a lot more confident and was breastfeeding more happily and that was fantastic.'

Reflect

How important is individual assessment when making an accurate judgement of factors that affect the woman's coping potential, such as level of nervousness, anxiety, confusion and self-efficacy? How consistent and caring are the advice and physical support that are given?

EXPRESSING BREAST MILK

In some instances, efforts to support positioning and attachment are hindered by anatomical difficulties in either the mother (due to flat or inverted nipples) or the infant (due to tongue tie). Where this occurs, it is crucial that milk production is stimulated successfully by expressing breast milk in order to stimulate prolactin production. Other physiological challenges can interfere with positioning and attachment, such as engorgement or mastitis, which will inhibit milk production if breast milk is not removed.

All breastfeeding mothers should be given information and be shown how to hand-express their breast milk. Milk expression may initially seem time-consuming and require a degree of patience, perseverance and dedication from the mother. The initial milk expression may only yield small volumes of milk, and reassurance should be given that this is normal when initiating lactation by milk expression. Verbal information and demonstrations should be reinforced by written information and reassurance about whom to turn to for help and advice in the longer term. Written information should be easy to read and the language should be user-friendly, as well as being sensitive to cultural differences and being translated into different languages, as appropriate.

Milk expression can also enable women to maintain their lactation throughout a period of planned or enforced separation. Although some separation may be enforced (e.g. due to illness), the majority of separation episodes will be planned for social and/or recreational reasons (e.g. in order to take planned breaks for shopping or enjoyment, to provide an opportunity for the father or others to feed the baby), or due to a return to employment.

Methods of milk expression

The Marmet technique is an internationally recognised method of hand expression which is effective in the first days of lactation, due to the thick consistency of colostrum, and when mature milk is produced.[110] Breast massage by nipple stimulation and breast handling before expression has been found to produce

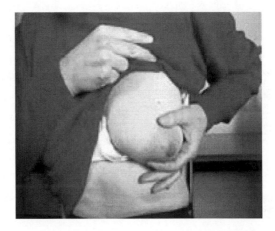

Using the thumb and forefinger, compress the lachterus sinuses in a steady rhythm.

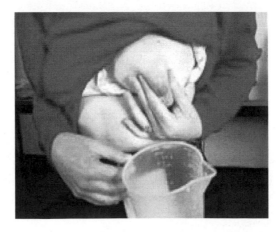

Milk may take a few minutes to flow. Rotate the fingers around the breast to empty all of the lobes.

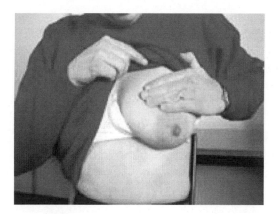

Stimulate the breast with massage.

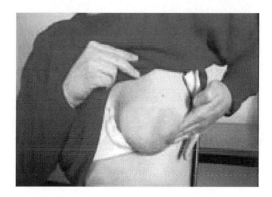

All around the breast.

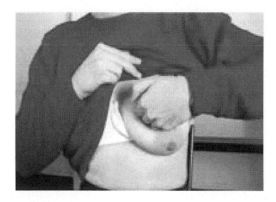

In whatever way mum wishes.

FIGURE 3.1: Hand expression (Reproduced with permission of the Chief Nursing Officer for Scotland).

a positive prolactin response.[111] Massage also promotes the release of oxytocin, which is required for milk ejection, and ensures that milk reservoirs are full before milk expression begins.

Breasts that are overfull may not release milk during expression, due to the effect of back pressure preventing the myo-epithelial cells from being contracted effectively by the hormone oxytocin. Application of warm cloths, warm showers and breast massage will all encourage the flow of breast milk throughout the breast. Furthermore, gentle hand expression may be more effective than a breast pump. Many mothers who need to express for longer or more frequently will choose to use a mechanical breast pump with a double pumping apparatus. The double pumping method of milk expression allows the simultaneous pumping of both breasts. This has been reported to stimulate higher serum prolactin levels, milk production and milk fat levels, and is often preferred by mothers because it takes less time.[112]

Storing and freezing human milk

Fresh breast milk can be kept at room temperature for up to 6 hours so long as it is stored in a sealed container.[113,114] Fresh breast milk can be stored in a refrigerator for 2 to 8 days at a temperature of 2–4 °C.[115,116] In a neonatal unit this storage time is reduced to 48 hours, due to the frequency of opening refrigerator doors to access stores.[117] Milk that has not been used after 48 hours should be frozen at −18°C for a maximum of 3 months, if it is to be fed to sick and/or preterm infants. If the infant is well, rather than discarding the milk at 3 months, it can be stored for a further 3 months. Breast milk can only be frozen in a freezer that has an appropriately high rating. Times vary for different types of freezer, and the manufacturer's instructions should be checked, but as a general rule, breast milk can be stored for the following times:

➤ 2 weeks in the freezer compartment of refrigerator
➤ 2 months in a refrigerator/freezer
➤ 6 months in a deep freeze maintained at −18°C or 0°F.

Thawing of breast milk

In order to avoid contamination, safety policies and procedures with regard to thawing of breast milk need to be in place, and appropriate safe information and guidance should be given to the mother. Breast milk must never be thawed and frozen again, nor should it be thawed or heated in a microwave oven, as some of the valuable properties are destroyed if it is heated to above 54.4°C. Heating in a microwave oven also creates hotspots which can scald.

Mothers who are expressing breast milk at home and transporting it to hospital should be advised of the different local and national recommendations for storage of milk in hospital. For example, the United Kingdom Association for Milk Banking provides guidelines for the collection, storage and handling of a mother's breast milk which is to be fed to her own baby on a neonatal unit.[118] Donor milk that is to be fed to another infant, rather than exclusively to a mother's own infant, is subject to stringent protocols, which vary from one country to another.

Thawed breast milk can be kept at room temperature for 1 hour or in a refrigerator for 24 hours. The correct method of thawing breast milk is to hold it initially under cold running water, gradually increasing the temperature of the running water. This process can take up to 10 minutes. An alternative method is to immerse the breast milk in a jug of hot water.

CONCLUSION

There is clear evidence that the implementation of Baby-Friendly practice standards results in consistency both of care and of information giving and guidance. However, despite this evidence, women who use maternity services continue to be subjected to differences in care, support, guidance and attitudes from healthcare professionals. Importantly, though, this is not always the case. There is growing recognition that the maternal experience has a profound and lasting effect on the experience of breastfeeding both at that time and in future pregnancies. The opportunity to challenge this situation has never been more open. All healthcare professionals have a professional obligation to be part of this very necessary change at a local level.

EXAMPLE: PRACTICE IMPROVEMENT PLAN

From the discussions in Chapters 2 and 3, the women's experiences of service provision have to be an integral part of any practice improvement plan. It is also important to highlight the fact that women can have a positive experience even when breastfeeding is unsuccessful, if there has been obvious help, encouragement and support offered. The template shown in Table 3.1 can be used by healthcare professionals to plan practice improvements and enhance local community services, particularly from the perspective of the users.

Each action point will be reviewed and updated. Implementation status monitored quarterly allows for identification of trouble spots and alternative actions required.

The template in Table 3.2 is an example of how improvements can be mapped out to enable reporting and accountability. Each area will have different needs which will be identified from the first two action points and then inform further actions which will contribute to efficient and effective use of resources and improve the experiences of breastfeeding women.

TABLE 3.1: Implementation status monitoring

Implementation status	Total (previous status in brackets)
√ Action completed	
J Action on course for completion	
X Little or no progress made	
? Not known, further information required	
↔ Change to action originally planned	
Ø Decision not to progress	

TABLE 3.2: Template for mapping improvements (objective: providing supportive and holistic care for breastfeeding mothers)

Action: postnatal community nursing	Lead	Team	Required	By when	Status	Measure (how much)
Explore staff views of barriers and opportunities to providing breastfeeding support to women and their families						
Explore mothers' views of early postnatal experience after discharge to health visitors (HVs)						
Review evidence and agree project definition, action plan, project plans, and tactical implementation plan						

FURTHER READING

NICE has produced guidelines on the implementation of Baby-Friendly practice standards. More information on these postnatal guidelines can be found on their website (http://guidance.nice.org.uk/CG37).

The Infant Feeding Survey 2000 was the sixth national survey in the UK looking at feeding practices for babies and infants and covering all countries of the UK.

It can be accessed on the UK Department of Health website (www.dh.gov.uk/en/Publicationsandstatistics/Publications/PublicationsStatistics/DH_4079223).

The UK Infant Feeding Survey for 2005 is also available online (www.ic.nhs.uk/statistics-and-data-collections/health-and-lifestyles-related-surveys/infant-feeding-survey/infant-feeding-survey-2005).

UNICEF and the UK Department of Health have produced an information leaflet, *Off to the Best Start*, which is available on the Baby-Friendly website (www.babyfriendly.org.uk/items/resource_detail.asp?item=455).

In Scotland, a website was developed for parents and healthcare professionals to help to support baby-led feeding. It covers a number of topics, and includes an excellent visual tool for correct positioning and attachment. This resource can be found on the NHS Scotland website (www.breastfeed.scot.nhs.uk/BabyLed/index.html).

The Baby-Friendly organisation has also produced a resource entitled *Breastfeeding Your Baby*, which contains useful information to help new mothers with breastfeeding (www.babyfriendly.org.uk/pdfs/bfyb_english1.pdf).

The WHO has published a report about relactation, entitled *Relactation: a review of experience and recommendations for practice*. This document is summarised and can be downloaded from the WHO website (www.who.int/child_adolescent_health/documents/who_chs_cah_98_14/en).

The Breastfeeding Network offers guidance on expressing and storing breast milk. This can be found on their website (www.breastfeedingnetwork.org.uk/pdfs/BFNExpressing&Storing.pdf).

REFERENCES

1 Dalzell J. *Exploring the infant feeding experiences of low-income mothers and the support offered by health professionals involved in their care: a qualitative study.* University of Dundee; 2007. Unpublished.
2 World Health Organization. *Protecting, Promoting and Supporting Breastfeeding: the role of maternity services.* Geneva: World Health Organization; 1989.
3 World Health Organization. *Innocenti Declaration on the Protection, Promotion and Support of Breastfeeding.* Geneva: World Health Organization; 1991.
4 Taveras EM, Li R, Grummer-Strawn L *et al.* Opinions and practices of clinicians associated with continuation of exclusive breastfeeding. *Pediatrics.* 2004; **113**: 283–90.
5 Guise JM, Palda V, Westhoff C *et al.* The effectiveness of primary care-based interventions to promote breastfeeding: systematic evidence review and meta-analysis by the US Preventive Services Task Force. *Ann Fam Med.* 2003; **1**: 70–78.

6 Gau ML. Evaluation of a lactation intervention program to encourage breastfeeding: a longuitudinal study. *Int J Nurs Stud.* 2004; **41:** 425–35.

7 Palmer G. *The Politics of Breastfeeding.* London: Pandora; 1993.

8 Winikoff B, Myers D, Laukaran VH *et al.* Dynamics of infant feeding: mothers, professionals, and the institutional context in a large urban hospital. *Pediatrics.* 1987; **80:** 423–33.

9 Garforth S, Garcia J. Breastfeeding policies in practice – 'No wonder they get confused.' *Midwifery.* 1989; **5:** 75–83.

10 Rajan L. The contribution of professional support, information and consistent advice to successful breastfeeding. *Midwifery.* 1993; **9:** 197–209.

11 UNICEF/WHO. *The UNICEF Baby-Friendly Hospital Initiative: ten steps to successful breastfeeding.* New York: UNICEF; 1992.

12 UNICEF. *Baby-Friendly Initiative: a seven point plan for the protection, promotion and support of breastfeeding in community health settings.* London: UNICEF; 1999.

13 World Health Organization. *Protecting, Promoting and Supporting Breastfeeding: the role of maternity services,* op. cit.

14 UNICEF/WHO. *The UNICEF Baby-Friendly Hospital Initiative: ten steps to successful breastfeeding,* op. cit.

15 UNICEF. *Baby-Friendly Initiative: a seven point plan for the protection, promotion and support of breastfeeding in community health settings,* op. cit.

16 Britten J, Broadfoot M. Breastfeeding support in Scotland. *Br J Midwifery.* 2002; **10:** 292–6.

17 Hamlyn B, Brooker S, Oleinkova K *et al. Infant Feeding 2000.* London: The Stationery Office; 2002. www.dh.gov.uk/en/Publicationsandstatistics/Publications/PublicationsStatistics/DH_4079223 (accessed 20 October 2009).

18 National Institute for Health and Clinical Excellence. *Postnatal Care: routine postnatal care of women and their babies.* NICE Guideline 37. London: National Institute for Health and Clinical Excellence; 2006. www.nice.org.uk/guidance/CG037

19 Akre J. Infant feeding: the physiological basis. *Bull World Health Organ.* 1989; **67:** 1–108.

20 Yokoyama Y, Ueda T, Irahara M *et al.* Releases of oxytocin and prolactin during breast massage and suckling in puerperal women. *Eur J Obstet Gynecol Reprod Biol.* 1994; **53:** 17–20.

21 Akre J, op. cit.

22 Slome C. Nonpuerperal lactation in grandmothers. *J Pediatr.* 1956; **39:** 45–8.

23 Wieschhoff H. Artificial stimulation of lactation in primitive cultures. *Bull Hist Med.* 1940; **8:** 1403–15.

24 Abejide OR, Tadese MA, Babajide DE *et al.* Non-puerperal induced lactation in a Nigerian community: case reports. *Ann Trop Paediatr Int Child Health.* 1997; **17:** 109–14.

25 Nemba K. Induced lactation: a study of 37 non-puerperal mothers. *J Trop Pediatr.* 1994; **40:** 240–42.

26 Gromada KK, Spangler AK. Breastfeeding twins and higher-order multiples. *J Obstet Gynecol Neonatal Nurs.* 1998; **27:** 441–9.

27 Perez-Escamilla R, Cohen RJ, Brown KH *et al.* Maternal anthropometric status and lactation performance in a low-income Honduran population: evidence for the role of infants. *Am J Clin Nutr.* 1995; **61:** 528–34.

28 Prentice AM, Roberts SB, Prentice A *et al.* Dietary supplementation of lactating Gambian women. I. Effect on breast-milk volume and quality. *Hum Nutr Clin Nutr.* 1983; **37**: 53–64.

29 Biancuzzo M. Breastfeeding multiples. *Childbirth Instructor.* 1998; **8**: 10–13.

30 Gromada KK, Spangler AK, op. cit.

31 Hartmann PE, Kent JC. The subtlety of breast milk. *Breastfeed Rev.* 1988; **13**: 14–18.

32 Ibid.

33 Akre J, op. cit.

34 Varendi H, Porter RH, Winberg J. Does the newborn find the nipple by smell? *Lancet.* 1994; **344**: 989–90.

35 Varendi H, Porter RH. Breast odour as the only maternal stimulus elicits crawling towards the odour source. *Acta Paediatr.* 2001; **90**: 372–5.

36 Bushnell JWR, Sai F, Mullin JT. Neonatal recognition of the mother's face. *Br J Dev Psychol.* 1989; **7**: 3–15.

37 Fifer WP, Moon CM. The role of the mother's voice in the organization of brain function in the newborn. *Acta Paediatr.* 1994; **397**: 86–93.

38 Christensson K, Cabrera T, Christensson E *et al.* Separation distress call in the human neonate in the absence of maternal body contact. *Acta Paediatr.* 1995; **84**: 468–73.

39 Moore ER, Anderson GC, Bergman N. Early skin-to-skin contact for mothers and their healthy newborn infants. *Cochrane Database Syst Rev.* 2007; **3**: CD003519.

40 Mikiel-Kostyra K, Mazur J, Boltruszko I. Effect of early skin-to-skin contact after delivery on duration of breastfeeding: a prospective study. *Acta Paediatr.* 2002; **91**: 1301–6.

41 De Chateau P, Wiberg B. Long-term effect on mother–infant behaviour of extra contact during the first hour postpartum. *Acta Paediatr.* 1977; **66**: 145–51.

42 Charpak N, Ruiz-Pelaez JG, Zita F *et al.* A randomized controlled trial of kangaroo mother care: results of follow-up at 1 year of corrected age. *Pediatrics.* 2001; **108**: 1072–9.

43 World Health Organization. *Kangaroo Mother Care: a practical guide.* Geneva: World Health Organization; 2003.

44 Christensson K, Cabrera T, Christensson E *et al.*, op. cit.

45 Bauer J. Metabolic rate and energy balance in the very low birth weight infants during kangaroo holding by their mothers and fathers. *J Pediatr.* 1996; **129**: 608–11.

46 Fohe K. Skin-to-skin contact improves gas exchange in premature infants. *J Perinatol.* 2000; **20**: 311–15.

47 Moore ER, Anderson GC, Bergman N, op. cit.

48 World Health Organization. *Kangaroo Mother Care: a practical guide,* op. cit.

49 Righard L, Alade MO. Breastfeeding and the use of pacifiers. *Birth.* 1990; **24**: 116–20.

50 Nissen E. Effects of maternal pethidine on infants' developing breastfeeding behaviour. *Acta Paediatr.* 1995; **84**: 140–45.

51 Rajan L. The impact of obstetric procedures and analgesia/anaesthesia during labour and delivery on breastfeeding. *Midwifery.* 1994; **10**: 87–103.

52 Nissen E, op. cit.

53 Woolridge MW. The 'anatomy' of infant sucking. *Midwifery.* 1986; **2**: 164–71.

54 Long L. Breastfeeding workshops: a focus on knowledge, skills and attitudes. *Br J Midwifery.* 1995; **3**: 540–42.

55 Renfrew MJ, Dyson L, Wallace L *et al. The Effectiveness of Public Health Interventions to Promote the Duration of Breastfeeding: systematic review.* London: National Institute

for Health and Clinical Excellence; 2005. www.nice.org.uk/page.aspx?o=511622 (accessed 5 October 2009).

56 McInnes RJ, Love JG, Stone DH. Evaluation of a community-based intervention to increase breastfeeding prevalence. *J Public Health Med.* 2000; **22**: 138–45.

57 Ballard JL, Auer CE, Khoury JC. Ankyloglossia: assessment, incidence, and effect of frenuloplasty on the breastfeeding dyad. *Pediatrics.* 2002; **110**: 63.

58 Fitz-Desorgher R. All tied up. Tongue tie and its implications for breastfeeding. *Pract Midwife.* 2003; **6**: 20–22.

59 Masaitis NS, Kaempf JW. Developing a frenotomy policy at one medical centre: a case study approach. *J Hum Lact.* 1996; **12**: 229–32.

60 Renfrew MJ, Dyson L, Wallace L et al., op. cit.

61 Enkin M, Keirse MJNC, Renfrew M et al. *A Guide to Effective Care in Pregnancy and Childbirth,* 2nd edn. Oxford: Oxford University Press; 1995.

62 Wylie J, Verber I. Why women fail to breast-feed: a prospective study from booking to 28 days post-partum. *J Hum Nutr Dietetics.* 1994; **7**: 115–20.

63 Hamlyn B, Brooker S, Oleinkova K et al., op. cit.

64 Morse JM, Jehle C, Gamble D. Initiating breastfeeding: a world survey of the timing of postpartum breastfeeding. *Breastfeed Rev.* 1992; **2**: 210–16.

65 Davies-Adetugbo AA. Sociocultural factors and the promotion of exclusive breast-feeding in rural Yoruba communities of Osun State, Nigeria. *Soc Sci Med.* 1997; **45**: 113–25.

66 Leefsman M, Habatsky T. The influence of hospital routine on successful breast-feeding. In: Frier S, Eidelman A (eds) *Human Milk: its biological and social value.* Amsterdam: Excerpta Medica; 1980. pp. 309–13.

67 Martin-Calama J, Buftuet J, Valero MJ et al. The effect of feeding glucose water to breastfeeding newborns on weight, body temperature, blood glucose and breastfeed-ing duration. *J Hum Lact.* 1997; **13**: 209–13.

68 Kurinij N, Shiono PH. Early formula supplementation of breastfeeding. *Pediatrics.* 1991; **88**: 745–50.

69 Feinstein JM, Berkelhamer JE, Gruszka ME et al. Factors related to early termination of breastfeeding in an urban population. *Pediatrics.* 1986; **78**: 210–15.

70 Blomquist HK, Jonsbo F, Serenius F et al. Supplementary feeding in the maternity ward shortens the duration of breastfeeding. *Acta Paediatr.* 1994; **83**: 1122–6.

71 Neifert MR, Seacat JM. Lactation insufficiency: a rational approach. *Birth.* 1987; **14**: 182–8.

72 Host A, Husby S, Osterballe O. A prospective study of cow's milk allergy in exclu-sively breastfed infants. Incidence, pathogenic role of early inadvertent exposure to cows' milk formula, and characterization of bovine milk protein in human milk. *Acta Paediatr Scand.* 1988; **77**: 66–70.

73 Atherton DJ, Sewell M, Soothill JF et al. A double-blind controlled crossover trial of an antigen-avoidance diet in atopic eczema. *Lancet.* 1978; **1**: 401–3.

74 Burr ML, Limb ES, Maguire MJ et al. Infant feeding, wheezing, and allergy: a prospec-tive study. *Arch Dis Child.* 1993; **68**: 724–8.

75 World Health Organization. *The International Code of Marketing of Breast-Milk Substitutes.* 1981. www.ibfan.org/site2005/Pages/article.php?art_id=52&iui=1 (accessed 5 October 2009).

76 Palmer B. The influence of breastfeeding on the development of the oral cavity: a commentary. *J Hum Lact.* 1998; **14**: 93–8.

77 Powers NG, Naylor AJ, Wester RA. Hospital policies: crucial to breastfeeding success. *Semin Perinatol.* 1994; **18**: 517–24.

78 Yamauchi Y, Yamanouchi I. Breastfeeding frequency during the first 24 hours after birth in full-term neonates. *Pediatrics.* 1990; **85**: 171–5.

79 Lindenberg CS, Artola RC, Jimenez V. The effect of early post-partum mother–infant contact and breastfeeding promotion on the incidence and duration of breastfeeding. *Int J Nurs Stud.* 1990; **27**: 179–86.

80 Buxton KE, Gielen AC, Faden RR *et al.* Women intending to breastfeed: predictors of early infant feeding experiences. *Am J Prev Med.* 1991; **7**: 101–6.

81 Keefe MR. The impact of infant rooming-in on maternal sleep at night. *J Obstet Gynecol Neonatal Nurs.* 1988; **17**: 122–6.

82 Bennett DE, Slade P. Reactions of mothers of preterm infants. *Midwife Health Visit Community Nurse.* 1990; **26**: 323–6.

83 Graham S. Psychological needs of families with babies in the neonatal unit: the role of the neonatal nurse. *J Neonatal Nurs.* 1995; **1**: 15–18.

84 McKim EM. The information and support needs of mothers of premature infants. *J Pediatr Nurs.* 1993; **8**: 233–44.

85 McKim E, Kenner C, Flandermeyer A *et al.* The transition to home for mothers of healthy and initially ill newborn babies. *Midwifery.* 1995; **11**: 184–94.

86 McHaffie H. Mothers of very low birthweight babies: how do they adjust? *J Adv Nurs.* 1990; **15**: 6–11.

87 McFadyen A. *Special Care Babies and their Developing Relationships.* London: Routledge; 1994.

88 Jaegar MC, Lawson M, Filteau S. The impact of prematurity and neonatal illness on the decision to breastfeed. *J Adv Nurs.* 1997; **25**: 729–37.

89 Keefe MR, op. cit.

90 Lemons JA, Moye L, Hall D *et al.* Differences in the composition of preterm and term human milk during early lactation. *Pediatr Res.* 1982; **16**: 113–17.

91 Lucas A, Morley R, Cole TJ *et al.* Breast milk and subsequent intelligence quotient in children born preterm. *Lancet.* 1992; **339**: 261–4.

92 Schanler RJ. Suitability of human milk for the low-birthweight infant. *Clin Perinatol.* 1995; **22**: 207–22.

93 Schanler R, Huist N. Human milk for hospitalised preterm infants. *Semin Perinatol.* 1994; **18**: 476–84.

94 Hopkinson JM, Schanler RJ, Garza C. Milk production by mothers of premature infants. *Pediatrics.* 1988; **81**: 815–19.

95 Kenner C, Lott J. Parent transition after discharge from the NICU. *Neonatal Netw.* 1990; **9**: 31–7.

96 Howard CR, Howard FM, Lanphear B *et al.* Randomized clinical trial of pacifier use and bottle-feeding or cup-feeding and their effect on breastfeeding. *Pediatrics.* 2003; **111**: 511–18.

97 Barros FC, Victoria CG. Use of pacifiers is associated with decreased breastfeeding duration. *Pediatrics.* 1995; **95**: 497–9.

98 Kramer MS, Barr RG, Dagenais S *et al.* Pacifier use, early weaning, and cry/fuss behaviour: a randomized controlled trial. *JAMA.* 2001; **286**: 322–6.

99 Newman J. Breastfeeding problems associated with early introduction of bottles and pacifiers. *J Hum Lact.* 1990; **6**: 59–63.

100 Wilson-Clay B, Brigham M. Clinical use of silicone nipple shields. *J Hum Lact.* 1996; **12:** 279–85.

101 Righard L, Alade MO, op. cit.

102 Auerbach KG. The effect of nipple shields on maternal milk volume. *J Obstet Gynecol Neonatal Nurs.* 1990; **19:** 419–27.

103 Ibid.

104 Neifert MR, Seacat JM, op. cit.

105 Lang S, Lawrence CJ, Orme RL. Cup feeding: an alternative method of infant feeding. *Arch Dis Child.* 1994; **71:** 365–9.

106 Stine MJ. Breastfeeding the premature newborn: a protocol without bottles. *J Hum Lact.* 1990; **6:** 167–70.

107 Kurokawa J. Finger-feeding a preemie. *Midwifery Today Childbirth Educ.* 1994; **spring issue:** 39.

108 Malhotra N, Vishwambaran L, Sundaram KR *et al.* A controlled trial of alternative methods of oral feeding in neonates. *Early Hum Dev.* 1999; **54:** 29–38.

109 Collins CT, Makrides M, Gillis J *et al.* Avoidance of bottles during the establishment of breast feeds in preterm infants. *Cochrane Database Syst Rev.* 2008; **4:** CD005252.

110 Mohrbacher N, Stock J. *The Breastfeeding Answer Book,* 3rd edn. Schaumburg, IL: La Leche League International; 2003.

111 Hopkinson JM, Schanler RJ, Garza C, op. cit.

112 Zinaman M, Hughes V, Queenan JT *et al.* Acute prolactin and oxytocin responses and milk yield to infant suckling and artificial methods of expression in lactating women. *Pediatrics.* 1992; **89:** 437–41.

113 Minder W, Roten H, Zurbrugg RP *et al.* Quality of breast milk: its control and preservation. *Helv Paediatr Acta.* 1982; **37:** 115–37.

114 Nwanko MU, Offor R, Okolo AA *et al.* Bacterial growth in expressed breast milk. *Ann Trop Paediatr Int Child Health.* 1988; **8:** 92–5.

115 Larson E, Zuill R, Zier V *et al.* Storage of human breast milk. *Infect Control.* 1984; **5:** 127–30.

116 Pardou A, Serruys E, Mascart-Lemone F *et al.* Human milk banking: influence of storage processes and bacterial contamination on some milk components. *Biol Neonate.* 1994; **65:** 302–9.

117 UK Association for Milk Banking. *Guidelines for the Collection, Storage and Handling of Mother's Breast Milk to be Fed to her Own Baby on a Neonatal Unit.* London: UK Association for Milk Banking; 2001.

118 Ibid.

CHAPTER 4

Supporting the continuation of breastfeeding

I was at the home of a friend's mum, my brother brought in a friend and he made a nasty comment about me doing it just to get my chest out for the other men in the room, that was a real surprise and everyone felt bad. But it was just ignorance and it didn't bother me . . . it does make me feel that there is no place you can breastfeed comfortably, other than your own home.[1]

INTRODUCTION

Some women and babies adapt to breastfeeding with relative ease, and experience an uneventful and enjoyable journey. However, not all women find initiating or continuing with breastfeeding a straightforward matter, and both psychological and physical factors are associated with breastfeeding cessation.[2]

The previous chapters have demonstrated an intricate interplay between social and individual factors, and have shown that the dynamics of this interplay affect a woman's attitude to and ability to cope with establishing breastfeeding.[3] The evidence also points to a direct relationship between the promotion, initiation and continuation of breastfeeding, and to the fact that most mothers are not sufficiently well prepared to cope with the experience of breastfeeding, especially with the problems that they may encounter.[4] This challenge may be compounded by traditional hospital routines, which may delay the timing of the first breastfeed or restrict mother–infant contact during the first 72 hours after birth.[5–7]

This chapter continues to explore this complex and dynamic interplay between the needs of the mother, the baby, the family, the socio-politico-economic environment (both within and outside the family) and professional practices. All of these factors influence a woman's decision to continue or cease breastfeeding. Discussions on poor positioning and attachment continue from the previous chapter, and these factors are identified as the root causes of many of the physical problems, including engorgement and mastitis, that are experienced by mothers during the early weeks of breastfeeding. Correct positioning and attachment have therefore been identified as a preventative solution to many of these physical problems.[8] However, there are additional factors that need to be acknowledged as having a powerful influence on the individual mother and family context.

COMMONLY ENCOUNTERED CHALLENGES

Maternal factors associated with continuation of breastfeeding are directly linked to a willingness and ability to cope with common physiological and psychological challenges.[9,10] Coping ability is in turn closely linked to the concept of self-efficacy. Renfrew *et al.* found that the art of caring, offering reassurance and information giving were fundamentally important.[11] This finding supports other evidence relating to women's self- efficacy. Women with a high self-efficacy score were found to be more likely to be breastfeeding and doing so exclusively at 1 week and 4 months than mothers with a low self-efficacy score.[12] Furthermore, other studies have found that enhancing the mother's confidence in her ability to breastfeed is more important and effective in helping her to continue to breastfeed than focusing on interventions aimed at knowledge and management of problems.[13]

Careful observation, monitoring and recording may pre-empt and therefore prevent problems, and when problems do occur, proactive and judicious management should be employed to minimise the negative effects on the mother and baby. There are four commonly encountered problems, which are likely to occur in the early days and weeks of breastfeeding:

➤ breast engorgement or full breasts
➤ lactating mastitis
➤ breast thrush infection
➤ milk insufficiency.

There is already a wealth of breastfeeding management information available to healthcare professionals, much of which is accessible from the various references that are cited throughout this book. The principles of providing support and guidance can be enhanced by utilising careful and considered assessment of breastfeeding.

TAKING A LACTATION HISTORY

Where problems are encountered, it can be useful to pull together all of the information necessary to make an assessment, and to develop a plan in partnership with the mother.

When taking a lactation history, ask relevant questions and make no assumptions. In a qualitative review of the literature, building a good relationship was viewed as important to mothers. The supportive healthcare professionals were those whom mothers perceived to be encouraging, non-judgemental, sympathetic, patient and understanding, in contrast to those who displayed a more directive or authoritarian manner.[14] Examples of approaches that were cited as being unhelpful were 'taking over' the care of the baby, or giving a lot of encouragement without any practical advice. These approaches were not perceived as being beneficial, and this often also led to concerns about conflicting advice.

Lactation history guide

The questions set out below provide the basis of a semi-structured approach to taking a lactation history. The factors are not exhaustive, and healthcare professionals may consider adding to and adapting these outline questions, based on their own experience. Three professional competencies contribute to this semi-structured approach, namely effective communication skills, effective observation skills and effective listening skills.

The mother

➤ How long has the mother been breastfeeding?
➤ How was breastfeeding established?
➤ Were there any delays in feeding?
➤ How were these delays managed?
➤ Were there any problems with positioning and attachment?
➤ How were these problems managed?
➤ When did the mother feel changes in her breasts associated with milk coming in?
➤ What are the presenting signs and symptoms at this time?
➤ When did these changes occur?
➤ If pain is present, ask the mother to describe where it is, its onset and its duration.
➤ What advice has the mother already received from the healthcare professional(s) and from family members?
➤ Has the mother been well?
➤ Is her appetite affected in any way?
➤ Is the mother taking any medication, including over-the-counter, prescribed or other remedies?

The infant

➤ What gestation was the baby at birth?
➤ What type of delivery was experienced?
➤ Were there any complications with the delivery?
➤ What type of analgesia was used in labour?
➤ Has the baby been unwell?
➤ How old is the baby at the time of the history?
➤ What is the feeding pattern, including frequency and length of feeds?

➤ What feeding behaviour is observed (rooting, eagerness, alertness, listlessness, breathlessness, tongue extension)?

➤ Is the baby on any medication?

➤ How often does the baby pass urine and stools?

➤ What colour are the urine and stools?

➤ Is the baby being given other foods/drinks, and if so by what method(s)?

➤ Is a pacifier used for the baby?

➤ What has the baby's weight trend been like?

The family

➤ How much does the mother know about breastfeeding?

➤ Is the mother's partner supportive of breastfeeding?

➤ Is the mother's family supportive of breastfeeding?

➤ How much help does the mother receive?

The information collated from the history can then be used to plan a supportive approach to problem solving, and to provide a solution to the presenting signs and symptoms. The techniques and approaches described in Chapter 3 can be applied. Creating opportunities to share case discussions about management approaches, thereby sharing evidence for practice among the members of the healthcare team, can also be helpful.

FEELING SUPPORTED

If a mother has a positive attitude and confidence in her ability to breastfeed, and she has the support of her family network, breastfeeding is much more likely to be successful.[15] In Chapters 2 and 3 we discussed the range of other supportive interventions that influence the establishment and continuation of breastfeeding. There are tremendous pressures on women, from both family and friends, which influence positive and negative emotions and feelings about breastfeeding.

Practice expert

The following vignette demonstrates the pressures, confusion and concerns associated with one woman trying to be a 'good' mother, and the range of emotions with which women can be struggling. Clearly, the strong family support that she received at a time of stress and anxiety proved a positive source of comfort for this mother, and supported her to continue breastfeeding.

Vignette: The potential of breastfeeding promotion by empowering

'My husband had been away from home working for the week. S must have only been 3 months old. I went to pick up my husband from the train station and S had been crying in the car, in his car seat, and I couldn't get him out to feed him. We were so close to home. When we got home the electricity had gone off, so we had to go and buy electric tokens. I remember picking up S and sitting on the bed and sitting in the dark because I couldn't put the electric on, he was screaming. I remember sitting on our bed and putting him on to feed and as soon as he went on he was feeding and he was happy. But I was crying my head off thinking I am a failure and my mum wants me to feed him a bottle and she may be right. I can't be a good mother because I can't feed him. Then my mum came in and she asked "What are you crying for?", and I said "You didn't think I can feed him properly myself, you think I should give him a bottle." She said "I am only suggesting a bottle because I know you are tired and you need to rest, but if it bothers you that much, express some milk and let someone else give him a bottle. You have had a baby and your hormones are all over the place, and you are not a failure, you are a brilliant mother."'

Reflect

Clearly, the praise from her mother was extremely important and beneficial in helping this woman to cope. Consider whether women who are isolated or who do not have a strong family network require additional support from healthcare professionals to continue breastfeeding. If so, think about what the nature of that support and the associated services might be.

A number of studies have identified that mothers harbour thoughts of stopping or actually cease breastfeeding within the first 2 weeks.[16-18] In these studies, an unsettled baby is commonly confused with and interpreted by the mother as being due to her having insufficient milk. However, Isabella and Isabella assessed breastfeeding mothers at 48 hours after birth and found that a positive maternal attitude towards breastfeeding, effective family support and experience of mother–infant bonding were significant factors relevant to the possibility of continuing breastfeeding.[19] Other studies have highlighted the availability of support to ensure that the baby is positioned and attached at the breast correctly, and that an effective sucking technique is established.[20,21]

STABILITY AND CONSISTENCY FROM A FAMILY UNIT

The presence of a supportive partner is known to have a positive effect on a woman's decision to breastfeed.[22] However, not all women who wish to breastfeed or who are considering the possibility of doing so have a supportive partner, and many other women have supportive partners who are away from the family unit for substantial periods of time (e.g. those in the armed forces, some nightshift workers, offshore workers, and partners who are in prison). Therefore stability and consistency in the family unit cannot always be guaranteed, and this gap may need to be filled by health services. In many parts of the developing world, and in countries torn apart by war, families may also be faced with a range of infectious diseases such as malaria, cholera and HIV/AIDS. In some parts of the world, the prevalence of HIV/AIDS may mean that it is a grandmother who is the sole remaining support for the whole family. In the developed world, many communities have a predominance of nuclear rather than extended families. Some social and economic problems and dysfunctional family structures are of a global nature. The reality is that the majority of women will be part of a social support system which at best is an aberration of what is assumed to be normal.[23]

Practice expert

Many women will experience the effect of interruption to their milk supply due to well-intended offers of help by family members. The desire of other family members to feed the baby was described by one mother as a problem, and highlights the potential impact of this and its contribution to milk insufficiency. This mother's mother-in-law looked after her baby every Wednesday.

Vignette: The importance of good family support

'I would go out for a couple of hours to do the shopping and what have you, but it seems to be as soon as I am out the door the bottles are made up and he is given a bottle, so when I have come back home say from the doctor's, she [mother-in-law] had given him a bottle for some apparent reason, so I was only away for about half an hour, but in that time he had had a 5 ounce bottle, so he started being sick.'

'I find it difficult come the Thursday and the Friday because it takes me a few days to then rebuild my milk back up to what he needs, because on the Wednesday I have not fed him as much as I should have fed him, so I do find it a lot more difficult like this because he is on the bottle rather than just being solely breastfed. I think it would have been easier if he had been solely breastfed.'

Reflect

The family's lack of knowledge about how the milk supply works, and their lack of support for the mother's strong desire to breastfeed, resulted in this mother becoming concerned about her milk supply.

MILK INSUFFICIENCY

A major concern in relation to supporting the continuation of breastfeeding is that milk insufficiency is often misdiagnosed.[24] The term 'milk insufficiency' is a blanket term for a physiological state that has a relatively large number of underlying causes. Importantly, surveys representing views from several countries have identified milk insufficiency as the most common reason cited by women for breastfeeding cessation.[25-29]

Anxiety about meeting the baby's feeding needs

Many studies have identified that the reasons for cessation of breastfeeding are associated with the demands of the baby for extra feeds, or simply linked to a baby crying or being irritable.[30–32] Concerns about breastfeeding and milk sufficiency are consequently related.[33,34] High levels of anxiety about being able to meet the baby's feeding needs are mentioned in many studies, and despite being a fairly common occurrence, they represent an important influence on decisions to cease breastfeeding. Concerns about milk sufficiency in particular have been cited in a number of papers as a reason for stopping breastfeeding.[35–41]

In summary, Renfrew *et al.* noted that milk insufficiency is often misdiagnosed, and that these babies present with four key signs:[42]

➤ crying after feeds
➤ feeding for long periods
➤ changing sleep patterns
➤ gaining weight slowly,

TABLE 4.1: Assessment of milk insufficiency: maternal causes to be considered

Maternal causes	
Poor production	Diet
	Illness
	Fatigue, stress, anxiety
	Structural causes
	Prior chest wall/breast surgery
	Thyroid conditions
	Severe postpartum haemorrhage
	Oestrogen-based oral contraceptive
	Retained placental products
	Polycystic ovary syndrome
	Anaemia
	Use of supplements
	Use of pacifier
	Use of nipple shield
	Absense of lactogenesis 1
	Postnatal depression
	Alcohol
Poor let-down	Psychological factors
	Drugs
	Smoking

Genuine milk insufficiency requires careful management, and greater attention needs to be paid to the underlying causes of milk insufficiency, with due consideration given to the fact that it can have a psychological basis. A mother may therefore perceive that she does not have sufficient milk when levels are in fact adequate, because of low levels of confidence and/or negative family and social influences. Mothers in such circumstances will benefit greatly from the support of a trained peer worker to provide information, encouragement and reassurance.[43,44]

Key management principles for milk insufficiency consist of observing a breastfeed, taking a lactation history, and agreeing a plan of action. Consideration must also be given to any significant weight loss that requires paediatric assessment. In some instances, continued breastfeeding should be encouraged, with supplements to ensure growth.

Tables 4.1 and 4.2 can be used to help with the assessment of milk insufficiency.

Renfrew *et al.* identified five areas where there is a lack of evidence from practice, and further research on milk insufficiency is required:[45]

➤ different types of milk insufficiency
➤ intrapartum causes and management
➤ randomised controlled trials (RCTs) for populations at high risk of milk insufficiency
➤ research on the effectiveness of current treatment regimes
➤ effectiveness of self-help models.

TABLE 4.2: Assessment of milk insufficiency: infant causes to be considered

Infant causes	
Poor intake	Poor positioning and attachment
	Restricted feeding
	Disorganised suck
	Structural causes – cleft palate
	Prematurity
	Effect of labour and delivery medications
	Jaundice
Low net intake	Diarrhoea and vomiting
	Malabsorption
	Infection
High energy requirement	Central nervous system abnormality
	Cardiac abnormality
	Small for gestational age

Practice expert

Women also identify concerns about their milk supply at the time when they start to express breast milk, comparing and relating the volume of milk expressed to an inadequate milk supply.

Vignette: Concerns about milk supply

'Then he started using me as a comforter so he was latching on but he wasn't feeding, so I started expressing milk, but when I was expressing milk I wasn't expressing enough for what he needed, so I started him on a mixture of formula as well and he was feeding off the formula, so I eventually dried up.'

'He was taking 6 ounces at 4 weeks, and I was letting myself fill up and then expressing it, and I was getting maybe 4 ounces out of both sides to make up a bottle, so I wasn't making enough to feed him and express it off as well, so I put him on the bottle and he settled down really well, so now he is feeding every two and a half hours.'

Reflect

The concerns highlighted by perception of insufficient volume require careful management and advice. Effective information giving is required to address this commonly held concern among breastfeeding mothers.

An additional management challenge of true milk insufficiency may be the potential or actual faltering growth of the infant. The elements of the problem must be identified as quickly as possible by taking a good lactation history, which will help to locate the key maternal and infant root causes.[46] Growth charts continue to be relied upon as a useful tool for assessing a baby's growth. However, they must be regarded as a reference point only, and not as a standard for growth. This is particularly so in breastfed babies, as research suggests that exclusively breastfed babies may display inconsistent growth patterns, with rapid growth in the first 3 months and a slower rate of growth from 4 to 12 months.[47,48] Growth charts therefore do not take into account the fact that infants have varying rates of growth and that they should be assessed on an individual basis.

There is increasing recognition in the UK and the USA that the growth charts currently in use are inappropriate for breastfed babies, and may even indicate or imply (inaccurately) faltering growth at 8 weeks.[49] Weight gain in breastfed infants slows down between 3 and 5 months, and professional advice should be supportive and reflect this evidence.[50] Weight charts based on a sample of 120 British, long-term breastfed infants from one geographical area have been developed by the Child Growth Foundation.[51] The WHO has completed the development of international growth standards for breastfed infants. Across the UK, introduction of this significant change began in 2009–10.

SOCIAL NETWORK SUPPORT AND PUBLIC SUPPORT FOR BREASTFEEDING

In a review of the qualitative literature, it was found that social network support may influence the mother's breastfeeding experience, and there was some evidence that mothers can be undermined by lack of knowledge within their social network, or by negative attitudes and beliefs.[52] Women with a supportive family network appeared to be more likely to overcome initial feeding difficulties than those whose families were not supportive. Unsupportive networks often left mothers feeling pressurised to change their behaviour. These mothers identified external support from peers or groups as being important to successful breastfeeding.[53]

Knowing that reliable and consistent support is available appears to be a relevant factor in alleviating anxiety. However, support can also be a factor in determining whether mothers decide to stop breastfeeding. In a study of mothers in England, it was found that the offer of regular childcare support by other female relatives was a predictor of early cessation of breastfeeding.[54] Kirkland and Fein also found that breastfeeding cessation was more likely to occur when the mother expressed an interest in being able to leave the infant with someone else, or in wanting another person to feed the baby.[55] The solution to these situations is for mothers to learn to express breast milk as soon as possible, and for breastfed babies to have the opportunity to become accustomed to receiving breast milk through a feeding cup.[56,57]

In Chapter 2 we discussed the introduction of the Scottish Parliamentary Bill that made it an offence to stop a mother breastfeeding in public. Although this type of legislative action goes some way towards empowering women to feel comfortable about breastfeeding in public, there are still significant barriers to this practice in reality, as demonstrated by the following accounts.

Preparing women adequately to cope with the various social reactions, values and attitudes that they will encounter with regard to breastfeeding in public is fundamental to supporting the continuation of breastfeeding. Adequate preparation goes a long way towards dealing with such issues.

Vignette: Changing social values

'His [her partner's] friends didn't want to visit in case I was breastfeeding.'

'At first you can't do it in front of people, so I used to take her upstairs, it was boring, but I never had confidence breastfeeding in front of loads of people. A woman told me the first three weeks are the worst. I felt if I could stick it for the three weeks I would manage.'

'My mum . . . she thinks it's really good, and my dad is really chuffed, but they aren't sitting in the room when I am doing it, but they have all been good.'

'I felt it was quite funny. My friends were so aware of me breastfeeding and maybe a touch embarrassed. It made them feel more comfortable to put me in another room when I went to visit them.'

'Obviously we did go out. It does crack you up staying at home all the time. For me there was no other way to settle him. If I was walking into town, just to the bottom of the road, that is a long way to go with a baby screaming. He wouldn't settle with a dummy [comforter], so it wasn't like he would take that and that would control him. There was a list of places that the health visitor gave me that made you aware of where you can breastfeed. A woman in the bed across from me in hospital said that she got thrown out of a canteen for breastfeeding.'

'My brother-in-law leaves the room when I start breastfeeding.'

'I was at the home of a friend's mum. My brother brought in a friend and he made a nasty comment about me doing it just to get my chest out for the other men in the room. That was a real surprise and everyone felt bad. But it was just ignorance, and it didn't bother me. It does make me feel that there is no place you can breastfeed comfortably, other than your own home.'

Reflect

Consider whether assessment processes and communication systems encourage and enable women to discuss the social issues associated with breastfeeding. Do they provide opportunities for offering guidance on how to cope with the various reactions to breastfeeding that are encountered within society? How is this managed at a local practice level?

PSYCHOLOGICAL STATE OF THE MOTHER

In developed countries, postnatal depression affects 10–15% of women,[58] and it has a significant negative impact on breastfeeding duration, but may go undiagnosed. In a study that assessed the relationship between depressive symptoms and breastfeeding at 6 and 12 weeks postpartum, depressive symptoms occurring early in the postpartum period were found to lead to a lower prevalence of breastfeeding.[59] In addition, it has been found that mothers with a high score on the Edinburgh Postnatal Depression Scale are more likely to stop breastfeeding early[60] but, importantly, the depressive disorder generally precedes breastfeeding cessation.[61] This study highlights the importance of early detection and intervention in postnatal depression. It can therefore be concluded that, given timely and correct advice and appropriate management and support, mothers with postnatal depression should be able to continue breastfeeding.

An Australian study of a cohort of 1745 women reported that breastfeeding was initiated by 96% of the participants. It was found that 79% of the women were still breastfeeding at 2 months, 57% at 6 months, and 22% at 12 months. Of the 18% of participants who were diagnosed with postnatal depression, the onset of this disorder occurred before 2 months in 63% of cases. Early cessation of breastfeeding was found to be significantly associated with postnatal depression, and the onset of postnatal depression occurred before cessation of breastfeeding in most cases. The authors concluded that postnatal depression has a significant negative impact on breastfeeding duration, and that assistance with breastfeeding problems should be included in the management of postnatal depression.[62]

BREASTFEEDING AND COPING WITH OTHER CHILDREN

When breastfeeding, it can be difficult to cope with the demands of other children. Exchanging information about how this could be managed may make a difference to breastfeeding duration. Before breastfeeding, other children should be taken to the toilet, and it should be ensured that everyone has a drink, telephone, remote, books, toys, etc. to hand, as appropriate. When the mother is feeding, the older child or children can be entertained by reading a book, singing nursery rhymes, or watching a DVD, thus ensuring that the mother has time to sit and enjoy feeding. If the mother has a friendly neighbour who could help out at feeding times, this may be another option whereby others can be involved in supporting the mother. Emphasising to women that being a new mother again requires time and energy is crucial for these women's self-esteem.

DEMANDS OF WORK

Mothers may face additional demands associated with work that have also been found to influence decisions to cease breastfeeding. This is especially so if legal, social or economic requirements necessitate their returning to work 3 months after the baby's birth.[63–66]

ALCOHOL INTAKE

Alcohol that has been consumed passes freely into the mother's milk and may have a detrimental effect on the baby's organs, including the brain. Blood alcohol levels peak 30–60 minutes after consumption without food, or 60–90 minutes after consumption when taken with food.[67] There is no documented evidence on safe alcohol limits during breastfeeding.

SMOKING AND ASSOCIATED FACTORS

Smoking during pregnancy is a strong predictor of postnatal smoking. Around 25% of women who stop smoking during pregnancy resume the habit after childbirth.[68] Women who smoke are less likely to intend to breastfeed, so it cannot be assumed that the relationship between smoking and duration of breastfeeding is a physiological one.[69]

Smoking does not have a consistently negative physiological effect on lactation. The wide variation in breastfeeding rates among women who do smoke would appear to demonstrate that it is likely that psychosocial factors may also play a significant part in lower rates of breastfeeding in women who smoke compared with those who do not.[70]

In one study, researchers found that more than 60% of women who gave up smoking during pregnancy resumed smoking in the months following birth (50% by approximately 4 months postpartum). Most of those who began smoking again had a partner who smoked, and most were less likely to breastfeed for more than 6 weeks.[71] In one study, 40% of babies were rated as colicky (defined as 2 to 3 hours of 'excessive' crying) by mothers who smoked and breastfed, compared with 26% of babies who were breastfed by non-smokers.[72]

Maternal smoking has been linked to early weaning, lowered milk production, and inhibition of the milk ejection or 'let-down' reflex. Smoking also lowers prolactin levels in the blood. One study by Hopkinson *et al.* clearly suggests that cigarette smoking significantly reduces breast milk production at 2 weeks postpartum, from 514 ml per day in non-smokers to 406 ml per day in smoking mothers.[73]

In Scotland, data on smoking trends during pregnancy and the postnatal period are collected by health visitors and stored in a child health surveillance programme database.

THE USE AND ABUSE OF SOCIAL DRUGS

Several so-called 'social drugs' are known to affect the composition and production of breast milk. Amphetamines, marijuana, cocaine, heroin and phencyclidine impair milk production, alter milk composition, and have adverse short- and long-term effects on the infant.[74]

MEDICATION

Drugs should be avoided where possible if they are not medically indicated. In the UK, national online resources are available to all healthcare professionals for learning about and checking the suitability of medication for prescribing during lactation (www.ukmicentral.nhs.uk/drugpreg/guide.htm and www.nes.scot.nhs.uk/pharmacy/breastfeeding/index.html).

In general, healthcare professionals should adopt the following principles when prescribing for breastfeeding mothers.

➤ Avoid unnecessary drug use, and limit use of over-the-counter (OTC) products.
➤ Breastfeeding mothers should seek advice on the suitability of OTC products.
➤ Assess the benefit/risk ratio for both mother and infant.
➤ Avoid the use of drugs that are known to cause serious toxicity in adults or children.
➤ Drugs that are licensed for use in infants are not generally a hazard.
➤ Neonates (especially premature infants) are at greater risk from exposure to drugs via breast milk, because of their immature excretory functions and the consequent risk of drug accumulation.

➤ Choose a regimen and route of administration that present the minimum amount of drug to the infant.

➤ It is best to avoid long-acting preparations, especially for drugs that are likely to cause serious side-effects (e.g. antipsychotic agents), as it is difficult to time feeds to avoid significant amounts of the drug entering the breast milk.

➤ Multiple drug regimens may pose an increased risk, especially when adverse effects, such as drowsiness, are cumulative.

➤ Infants who are exposed to drugs via breast milk should be monitored for unusual signs or symptoms.

➤ Avoid the use of new drugs if a therapeutically equivalent alternative that has been more widely used is available. A robust assessment of the benefit/risk ratio requires data both on the passage of the drug into breast milk and on its effects in infants. There is rarely enough information available for new drugs to allow such an assessment to be made.

SUPPORTING MOTHERS
Peer support

With regard to giving new mothers confidence in the practical skill of breastfeeding, seeing someone else successfully breastfeed is more effective than being provided with theoretical information about the benefits.[75] A Cochrane Review also concluded that there is clear evidence of the effectiveness of lay support in promoting exclusive breastfeeding.[76] Although this finding may substantiate the setting up of peer support systems, the full effect of lay involvement in supporting women who are breastfeeding is as yet uncertain.[77]

Midwives and other professionals, as well as government organisations, are identified as leading the movement to de-medicalise pregnancy and childbirth.[78] The use of peer support as a strategy can be considered as a natural extension of this movement by recognising the value of women supporting women. The evidence suggests that peer support is an effective strategy for supporting women generally, and it has been shown to be effective during the antenatal and postnatal periods.[79] Furthermore, a positive relationship has been found between rates of continuation and contact with other breastfeeding mothers.[80-82] A Cochrane Review considered the value of extra support for breastfeeding mothers, beyond the usual care from health professionals and lay supporters, and concluded that consideration should be given to the setting up of additional support networks.[83]

⤴ Peer support is therefore associated with factors such as self-efficacy, and demonstrates the potential to politically empower women to become active in influencing and supporting breastfeeding practices. It also demonstrates that the involvement of women in helping other women to breastfeed is a model that warrants further exploration and research. There is also the possibility, which has yet to be explored thoroughly, that peer support strategies may embrace intimately the social, cultural and personal factors that are unique to each woman, and that peer support may be seen as a modern-day replacement for the traditional extended family support which has been lost, particularly in many developed countries. However, as a model, peer support may not be transferable to all cultures, and it may differ in character from one culture to another. An additional consideration is that studies to date have been conducted with study populations where breastfeeding is the norm rather than the exception.

Peer support is known to have a positive impact on breastfeeding self-efficacy, enabling the mother to continue with breastfeeding.[84,85] This also includes the development of different systems of lay support, including the use of role models.[86] Studies in the USA substantiate this finding, showing that peer support is particularly effective for women on a low income, and that it increases exclusive breastfeeding and the duration of breastfeeding.[87-89] In Scotland, a study of peer support for women on a low income found an increase in initiation rates, but unlike the US study did not show an increase in the duration of breastfeeding.[90]

Some peer support schemes have been developed with the aim of operating an antenatal apprenticeship scheme using mothers who have experienced success in breastfeeding. This, it is reasoned, will allow new mothers to acquire the practical skills of breastfeeding.[91] In this respect, peer support has been found to be beneficial for mothers with a low level of confidence, because it provides a structured environment in which they feel safe to express their personal concerns, knowing that they will receive support.[92] Taking such an approach will facilitate confidence building and the subsequent commitment of women to breastfeed. As with the other US and UK studies, Protheroe found this approach to be particularly effective with women who are on a low income.[93]

Given the health benefits and economic gains that are provided by breast-feeding for at least 6 months, peer support is undoubtedly an area that warrants further investment by governments and strategic planners.

A study based on a randomised controlled trial of a local peer support scheme, using the telephone, was conducted in Canada,[94] with experienced, successful breastfeeding women volunteers providing peer support for new mothers. The peer supporters initiated the contact with the breastfeeding mothers, with the aim of enabling the mothers to gain confidence to continue breastfeeding.

The results of this study demonstrated a significant increase in the number of mothers who breastfed until 3 months, and an increase in the number who breastfed exclusively.[95] The women in the intervention group were significantly more satisfied with their feeding experience, and were very satisfied with the peer support that they received. The authors of the study concluded that peer support increases both satisfaction levels and the potential for exclusive breastfeeding.

Professional support

As has already been mentioned, there has been increasing evidence over the last 50 years of successful political reaction to the medicalisation of pregnancy and childbirth, with the growing importance of the concept of normality in childbirth.[96] The Baby-Friendly standards provide direction for a range of healthcare professionals who provide support for breastfeeding. These standards include guidance for professionals on establishing breastfeeding support groups.

> Promote cooperation between healthcare staff, breastfeeding support groups and the local community.
>
> (Baby-Friendly practice standard)

Breastfeeding groups, baby cafés and early years groups can all offer additional support, peer support, and access to professional information and guidance, and they enable and support self-belief in breastfeeding mothers, which is so important for the continuation of breastfeeding.

In addition to locally run groups, there are a number of national support networks that offer breastfeeding support. They generally run telephone helplines as well as information websites. In the UK these are as follows:

➤ Association of Breastfeeding Mothers   www.abm.me.uk
➤ Breastfeeding Network   www.breastfeedingnetwork.org.uk
➤ La Leche League GB   www.laleche.org.uk
➤ National Childbirth Trust   www.nctpregnancyandbabycare. com/home

Changing attitudes and value systems

The global professional challenge to increase breastfeeding rates cannot be underestimated. It has already been mentioned that the health benefits of breastfeeding are acknowledged by bottle-feeding mothers and breastfeeding mothers alike.[97] However, the same study also established that the interpretation of convenience in feeding method differs in the two groups. An important conclusion from this study is that knowledge of the benefits of breastfeeding is not enough to persuade mothers to start and then continue breastfeeding, and that lifestyle factors and other practical and psychological factors have a substantial influence on a woman's final feeding choice. Furthermore, it has been found that peer support programmes are less effective for women who have already made the decision to bottle-feed.[98]

Monitoring the quality of the service provided

Underpinning all professional support there should be systems to monitor the quality and effectiveness of the service that is provided. This is fundamental to supporting mothers to continue breastfeeding. There is clear evidence that mothers require a certain level of support from a variety of sources, and having in place rigorous monitoring and support systems will substantially increase breastfeeding rates, as healthcare professionals are central to the success of such a system.[99-104]

Porteous *et al.* and Serafino-Cross and Donovan advise that immediate and ongoing postnatal care in the community should be provided by individuals who are knowledgeable and skilled in breastfeeding support.[105,106] This includes the use of peer support systems. However, professionals require the political and economic support of governments in order to put in place the required range of strategies. Policy and practice need to be creative and will depend on the economic and social situation of local populations. For example, writing a self-monitoring journal has been found to be beneficial in empowering mothers who live in disadvantaged communities, and is recognised as being a powerful intervention, resulting in a positive outcome when milk insufficiency occurs.[107]

REVIEWING TRADITIONAL PRACTICES

In reviewing current practice with the aim of ensuring best and evidence-based practice, it is important to bear in mind the old adage that we 'do not throw the baby out with the bath water.' A number of practices that are implemented in the hospital setting during the postnatal period have been evaluated positively as enhancing breastfeeding duration. These include:

➤ skilled proactive help for mothers who want to breastfeed[108,109]
➤ a policy of no formula advertising, which is recommended as part of the International Code of Marketing of Breast-Milk Substitutes, and should be part of a breastfeeding policy for those hospitals that are working towards Baby-Friendly Hospital status[110]
➤ baby-led feeding, which allows prolactin receptor sites to be primed and ensures a good milk supply[111]
➤ unrestricted skin-to-skin contact[112]
➤ giving supplementary fluids only when medically indicated[113]
➤ continuation of breastfeeding where mastitis is a problem, with support given to ensure that the affected breast is adequately drained, and antibiotic therapy prescribed if infective mastitis occurs.[114]

Renfrew *et al.* and others have identified certain aspects of professional practice, which women have experienced during pregnancy and the postnatal period, that are detrimental to breastfeeding duration.[115] These include the following:

➤ inappropriate preparation of nipples for lactation
➤ Hoffman exercises for inverted nipples
➤ using breast shells in pregnancy
➤ distribution of information leaflets without discussion of the leaflet content[116]
➤ general practitioner consultation at 1 week postpartum[117]
➤ only one home visit by a community nurse[118]
➤ dopamine antagonists being prescribed for insufficient milk[119]
➤ mothers being provided with an individual self-help manual[120]
➤ antenatal education being provided by a paediatrician[121]
➤ providing information materials on infant feeding that are produced by formula milk companies.[122]

CONCLUSION

There are a number of factors that affect the continuation of breastfeeding. Self-belief and self-efficacy play a major role in enabling women to breastfeed not only when there are physiological challenges, but also when there are attitudinal and cultural barriers within the woman's family or social context. Clearly the most important element throughout is support from all parts of the professional network, family, friends and the community. Consider how professionals contribute to this agenda and reflect on how small changes can make a real difference to women and their families. A fundamental premise for practice is that effective support has the potential to have a direct effect on local and national breastfeeding rates. However, success is predicated on women having continuous support to initiate and continue breastfeeding.

PRACTICE IMPROVEMENT

In Scotland, for example, breastfeeding is one of the seven health improvement targets identified by the Scottish Government. The overarching outcome or goal on the left-hand side of Table 4.3 is to 'Increase the proportion of newborn children exclusively breastfed at 6–8 weeks from 26.6% in 2006–07 to 33.3% in 2010–11.' To provide an informative link between the outcome and operations, the outcome is accompanied by drivers for accomplishing that outcome. In this example, five primary drivers have been identified in Table 4.3, namely reliable data collection systems, the use of evidence-based practice standards to optimise initiation of breastfeeding, the use of evidence-based practice standards to optimise continuation of breastfeeding, giving pregnant women and new mothers appropriate, reliable and timely care, and contributing to national strategy development. Each of the drivers is a goal assigned to one or more individuals, with its own set of secondary drivers. The person or group responsible for the primary driver is also responsible for establishing the set of associated secondary drivers.

A driver diagram can then be used to develop a comprehensive implementation plan involving projects specific to the secondary drivers. These can in turn be allocated to a responsible officer who is accountable for delivery of the plan. Fundamental to the improvement plan is the utilisation of women's experiences to inform service improvements for women by women.

FURTHER READING

The Breastfeeding Network provides an excellent resource for mothers on breastfeeding and thrush, and also addresses the problem of nipple pain (this can be accessed at www.breastfeedingnetwork.org.uk/thrush-and-breastfeeding.html).

The Breastfeeding Network also provides information about the signs of mastitis and its treatment (www.breastfeedingnetwork.org.uk/pdfs/BFN_Mastitis.pdf).

TABLE 4.3: Driver diagram for practice improvement

Outcomes	Primary driver		Secondary drivers
Increase the proportion of newborn children exclusively breastfed at 6–8 weeks from 26.6% in 2006–07 to 33.3% in 2010–11	Data collection systems for breastfeeding statistics are reliable and enable monitoring of H7 target at 6–8 week review	→	Shared clinical guidelines for data input and collection
			Optimise data collected for 'reason for stopping breastfeeding' field
	Maternity service staff and voluntary sector staff provide appropriate, reliable and timely care to pregnant women and new mothers using UK UNICEF evidence-based practice standards to optimise the initiation of breastfeeding	→	Optimise adherence to UK UNICEF Baby-Friendly hospital standards
			Create a culture that utilises volunteers to support new mothers
			Create a supportive, encouraging environment which prioritises breastfeeding support
			Optimise breastfeeding support by partners and significant others
	Community Health Partnership (CHP) staff provide appropriate, reliable and timely care to pregnant women and new mothers using UK UNICEF evidence-based practice standards to optimise the continuation of breastfeeding	→	Optimise adherence to UK UNICEF Baby-Friendly community standards
			Create a culture that utilises volunteers to support new mothers
			Optimise the support provided for community breastfeeding groups
			Create partnerships with other organisations which have contact with new families

(continued)

TABLE 4.3 (continued)

Outcomes		Primary driver		Secondary drivers
Increase the proportion of newborn children exclusively breastfed at 6–8 weeks from 26.6% in 2006–07 to 33.3% in 2010–11	→	Pregnant women and new mothers receive appropriate, reliable and timely care which complies with UK UNICEF evidence-based practice standards for initiation and continuation of breastfeeding	→	Create a better understanding of the reasons for breastfeeding decline at 6–8 week review
				Prioritise the preparation of pregnant women for breastfeeding
				Optimise support for the women most likely to stop breastfeeding
				Create a positive culture and attitude for the support of breastfeeding
	→	Contribute to National Infant Feeding Strategy for Scotland	→	Create a shared vision for improving breastfeeding initiation and continuation rates in Scotland
				Optimise breastfeeding promotional campaigns

For further information about mastitis, the WHO has a report available online, entitled *Mastitis: causes and management* (http://whqlibdoc.who.int/hq/2000/WHO_FCH_CAH_00.13.pdf).

Further information about HIV and breastfeeding is available online, and the WHO is a useful source of information and evidence on this topic (the 2009 revised principles and recommendations on infant feeding in the context of HIV can be found at www.who.int/child_adolescent_health/documents/9789241598873/en/index.html).

Information about mother-to-child transmission of HIV and publications relating to this topic can also be found on the WHO website (www.who.int/hiv/topics/mtct/en).

NHS Health Scotland provides online reports which are based on the work of the Breastfeeding Expert Group, which was set up to gather best evidence on breastfeeding which could support attempts to increase breastfeeding rates (these reports and the minutes of group meetings can be found at www.healthscotland.com/resources/networks/early-years/beg.aspx).

In 2002, the Scottish Intercollegiate Guidelines Network (SIGN) published *Postnatal Depression and Puerperal Psychosis: a national clinical guideline*. This offers clinicians guidance on preferred management practices for these conditions (and is available online at www.sign.ac.uk/guidelines/published/index.html#obstetrics).

It is important for healthcare professionals to be able to access reliable information about new and existing drugs and their use in lactating women (information about a range of medications can be found at www.ukmicentral.nhs.uk/drugpreg/guide.htm).

An online educational resource has been produced by NHS Education for Scotland which provides an e-learning programme of information and recommendations for prescribing during lactation. This is aimed at healthcare professionals (and can be found at www.nes.scot.nhs.uk/pharmacy/breastfeeding/index.html).

Healthcare professionals may need to give mothers information about weaning, and the Infant Dietetic Food Association provides information on this (available online at www.idfa.org.uk/sn_wn.aspx).

REFERENCES

1 Dalzell J. *Exploring the infant feeding experiences of low-income mothers and the support offered by health professionals involved in their care: a qualitative study.* University of Dundee; 2007. Unpublished.

2 Cooper PJ, Murray L, Stein A. Psychosocial factors associated with the early termination of breast-feeding. *J Psychosom Res.* 1993; **37**: 171–6.

3 Cernadas JM, Noceda G, Barrera L et al. Maternal and perinatal factors influencing the duration of exclusive breastfeeding during the first 6 months of life. *J Hum Lact.* 2003; **19**: 136–44.

4 Colin WB, Scott JA. Breastfeeding: reasons for starting, reasons for stopping and problems along the way. *Breastfeed Rev.* 2002; **10**: 13–19.

5 Dennis C, Hodnett E, Gallop R et al. The effect of peer support on breastfeeding duration among primiparous women: a randomized controlled trial. *Can Med Assoc J.* 2002; **166**: 21–8.

6 Lawson K, Tulloch MI. Breastfeeding duration: prenatal intentions and postnatal practices. *J Adv Nurs.* 1995; **22**: 841–9.

7 Wylie J, Verber I. Why women fail to breast-feed: a prospective study from booking to 28 days post-partum. *J Hum Nutr Dietetics.* 1994; **7**: 115–20.

8 Henderson A, Kitzinger J, Green J. Representing infant feeding: content analysis of British media portrayal of bottle feeding and breastfeeding. *BMJ.* 2000; **311**: 1196–8.

9 Cooper PJ, Murray L, Stein A, op. cit.

10 Cernadas JM, Noceda G, Barrera L et al., op. cit.

11 Renfrew MJ, Woolridge MW, Ross McGill H. *Enabling Women to Breastfeed: a review of practices which promote or inhibit breastfeeding – with evidence-based guidance for practice.* London: The Stationery Office; 2000.

12 Blythe R, Creedy D, Dennis CL et al. Effect of maternal confidence on breast-feeding duration: an application of breast-feeding self-efficacy theory. *Birth.* 2002; **29**: 278–84.

13 Ertem IO, Votto N, Leventhal JM. The timing and predictors of the early termination of breastfeeding. *Pediatrics.* 2001; **107**: 543–8.

14 McInnes RJ, Love JG, Stone DH. Evaluation of a community-based intervention to increase breastfeeding prevalence. *J Public Health Med.* 2000; **22**: 138–45.

15 Cernadas JM, Noceda G, Barrera L et al., op. cit.

16 Colin WB, Scott JA, op. cit.

17 Cooke M, Sheehan A, Schmied V. A description of the relationship between breast-feeding experiences, breastfeeding satisfaction, and weaning in the first 3 months after birth. *J Hum Lact.* 2003; **19**: 145–56.

18 Dykes F, Williams C. Falling by the wayside: a phenomenological exploration of perceived breast-milk inadequacy in lactating women. *Midwifery.* 1999; **15**: 232–46.

19 Isabella PH, Isabella RA. Correlates of successful breastfeeding: a study of social and personal factors. *J Hum Lact.* 1994; **10**: 257–64.

20 Cernadas JM, Noceda G, Barrera L et al., op. cit.

21 Isabella PH, Isabella RA, op. cit.

22 Basire K, Pullon S, McLeod D. Baby feeding: the thoughts behind the statistics. *N Z Med J.* 1997; **110**: 184–7.

23 Cernadas JM, Noceda G, Barrera L et al., op. cit.

24 Renfrew MJ, Dyson L, Wallace L et al. *The Effectiveness of Public Health Interventions*

to Promote the Duration of Breastfeeding: systematic review. London: National Institute for Health and Clinical Excellence; 2005. www.nice.org.uk/page.aspx?o=511622 (accessed 5 October 2009).

25 World Health Organization. *Report on the WHO Collaborative Study on Breastfeeding: contemporary patterns of breastfeeding.* Geneva: World Health Organization; 1981.

26 Akre J. Infant feeding: the physiological basis. *Bull World Health Organ.* 1989; **67 (Supplement):** 1–108.

27 White A, Freeth S, O'Brien M. *Infant Feeding 1990.* London: HMSO; 1992.

28 Foster K, Lader D, Cheesborough S. *Infant Feeding: a survey of infant feeding practices in the United Kingdom.* London: The Stationery Office; 1997.

29 Hamlyn B, Brooker S, Oleinkova K *et al. Infant Feeding 2000.* London: Department of Health; 2002. www.dh.gov.uk/en/Publicationsandstatistics/Publications/Publications Statistics/DH_4079223 (accessed 23 October 2009).

30 Bailey VF, Sherriff J. Reasons for the early cessation of breastfeeding in women from lower socio-economic groups in Perth, Western Australia. *Breastfeed Rev.* 1993; **2:** 390–3.

31 Matthews K, Webber K, McKim E *et al.* Maternal infant-feeding decisions: reasons and influences. *Can J Nurs Res.* 1998; **30:** 177–98.

32 Colin WB, Scott JA, op. cit.

33 Dykes F, Williams C, op. cit.

34 Britton C, McCormick F, Renfrew MJ *et al.* Support for breastfeeding mothers. *Cochrane Database Syst Rev.* 2007; **1:** CD001141.

35 Bailey VF, Sherriff J, op. cit.

36 Isabella PH, Isabella RA, op. cit.

37 Avery M, Duckett L, Dodgson J *et al.* Factors associated with very early weaning among primiparas intending to breastfeed. *Matern Child Health J.* 1998; **2:** 167–79.

38 Chen W. Perceived breast milk inadequacy was related to sociocultural influences and the behaviour of women and their babies. *Evid Base Nurs.* 2000; **3:** 131.

39 Colin WB, Scott JA, op. cit.

40 Kirkland VL, Fein SB. Characterizing reasons for breastfeeding cessation throughout the first year postpartum using the construct of thriving. *J Hum Lact.* 2003; **19:** 278–85.

41 Bolling K, Grant K, Hamlyn B *et al. Infant Feeding Survey 2005: a survey conducted on behalf of the Information Centre for Health and Social Care and the UK Health Departments.* London: BMRB Social Research; 2007.

42 Renfrew MJ, Dyson L, Wallace L *et al.,* op. cit.

43 Dennis C, Hodnett E, Gallop R *et al.,* op. cit.

44 Hoddinott P, Pill R. Qualitative study of decisions about infant feeding among women in east end of London. *BMJ.* 1999; **318:** 30–34.

45 Renfrew MJ, Dyson L, Wallace L *et al.,* op. cit.

46 Lawrence RA, Lawrence RM. *Breastfeeding: a guide for the medical profession,* 5th edn. St Louis, MO: Mosby; 1999.

47 Cohen RJ, Brown KH, Canahuati J *et al.* Effects of age introduction of complementary foods on infant breast milk intake, total energy intake, and growth: a randomised controlled study in Honduras. *Lancet.* 1994; **344:** 288–93.

48 Dewey KG, Peerson JM, Brown KH *et al.* Growth of breast-fed infants deviates from current reference data: a pooled analysis of US, Canadian, and European data sets.

World Health Organization Working Group on Infant Growth. *Pediatrics.* 1995; **96:** 495–503.

49 Cole TJ, Paul AA, Whitehead RG. Weight reference charts for British long-term breast-fed infants. *Acta Paediatr.* 2002; **91:** 1296–300.

50 Kramer MS, Guo T, Platt RW *et al.* Breastfeeding and infant growth: biology or bias? *Pediatrics.* 2002; **110:** 343–7.

51 Fry T. The new 'Breast from Birth' growth charts. *J Fam Health Care.* 2003; **13:** 124–6.

52 McInnes RJ, Love JG, Stone DH, op. cit.

53 Ibid.

54 Bick DE, MacArthur C, Lancashire RJ. What influences the uptake and early cessation of breastfeeding? *Midwifery.* 1998; **14:** 242–7.

55 Kirkland VL, Fein SB, op. cit.

56 Thapa S, Short R, Potts M. Breastfeeding, birth spacing and their effects on child survival. *Nature.* 1988; **335:** 679–82.

57 Deacon C. Whose breasts are they anyway? *New Generation.* 1998; **17**.

58 Tammentie T, Tarkka MT, Astedt_Kurki P *et al.* Family dynamics and postnatal depression. *Can J Nurs Res.* 2004; **11:** 141–52.

59 Hatton DC, Harrison-Hohner J, Coste S *et al.* Symptoms of postpartum depression and breastfeeding. *J Hum Lact.* 2005; **21:** 444–9.

60 Bick DE, MacArthur C, Lancashire RJ, op. cit.

61 Cooper PJ, Murray L, Stein A, op. cit.

62 Henderson JJ, Evans S, Straton JAY *et al.* Impact of postnatal depression on breast-feeding duration. *Birth.* 2003; **30:** 175–80.

63 Avery M, Duckett L, Dodgson J *et al.,* op. cit.

64 Bergh AM. Obstacles to and motivation for successful breastfeeding. *Curationis.* 1993; **16:** 24–9.

65 Bick DE, MacArthur C, Lancashire RJ, op. cit.

66 Matthews K, Webber K, McKim E *et al.* Maternal infant-feeding decisions: reasons and influences. *Can J Nurs Res.* 1998; **30:** 177–98.

67 Renfrew MJ, Dyson L, Wallace L *et al.,* op. cit.

68 Hamlyn B, Brooker S, Oleinkova K *et al.,* op. cit.

69 Amir LH. Maternal smoking and reduced duration of breastfeeding: a review of possible mechanisms. *Early Hum Dev.* 2001; **64:** 45–67.

70 Amir LH, Donath SM. Does maternal smoking have a negative physiological effect on breastfeeding? The epidemiological evidence. *Birth.* 2002; **29:** 112–23.

71 Mullen PD, Richardson MA, Quinn VP *et al.* Postpartum return to smoking: who is at risk and when. *Am J Health Promot.* 1997; **11:** 323–30.

72 Matheson I, Rivrud GN. The effect of smoking on lactation and infantile colic. *JAMA.* 1989; **261:** 42–3.

73 Hopkinson JM, Schanler RJ, Fraley K *et al.* Milk production by mothers of premature infants: influence of cigarette smoking. *Pediatrics.* 1992; **90:** 934–8.

74 Renfrew MJ, Dyson L, Wallace L *et al.,* op. cit.

75 Hoddinott P, Pill R, op. cit.

76 Britton C, McCormick F, Renfrew MJ *et al.,* op. cit.

77 Ibid.

78 Johanson R, Newburn M. Promoting normality in childbirth. *BMJ.* 2001; **323:** 1142–3.

79 Protheroe L, Dyson L, Renfrew M. *The Effectiveness of Public Health Interventions to Promote the Initiation of Breastfeeding.* Evidence Briefing. London: Health Development Agency; 2003.

80 Bergh AM, op. cit.

81 Hoddinott P, Pill R, op. cit.

82 Basire K, Pullon S, McLeod D, op. cit.

83 Britton C, McCormick F, Renfrew MJ *et al.,* op. cit.

84 Dennis C, Hodnett E, Gallop R *et al.,* op. cit.

85 Hoddinott P, Pill R, op. cit.

86 Britton C, McCormick F, Renfrew MJ *et al.,* op. cit.

87 Arlotti JP, Cottrell BH, Lee SH *et al.* Breastfeeding among low-income women with and without peer support. *J Community Health Nurs.* 1998; **15:** 163–78.

88 Schafer E, Vogel MK, Viegas S *et al.* Volunteer peer counsellors increase breastfeeding duration among rural low-income women. *Birth.* 1998; **25:** 101–6.

89 Kirstin N, Abramson R, Dublin P. Effect of peer counsellors on breastfeeding initiation, exclusivity and duration among low-income women. *J Hum Lact.* 1994; **10:** 11–15.

90 McInnes RJ, Love JG, Stone DH, op. cit.

91 Hoddinott P, Pill R, op. cit.

92 Protheroe L, Dyson L, Renfrew M, op. cit.

93 Ibid.

94 Dennis C, Hodnett E, Gallop R *et al.,* op. cit.

95 Ibid.

96 Johanson R, Newburn M, op. cit.

97 Zimmerman DR, Guttman N. 'Breast is best': knowledge among low-income mothers is not enough. *J Hum Lact.* 2001; **17:** 14–19.

98 Protheroe L, Dyson L, Renfrew M, op. cit.

99 World Health Organization, op. cit.

100 Akre J, op. cit.

101 White A, Freeth S, O'Brien M, op. cit.

102 Foster K, Lader D, Cheesborough S, op. cit.

103 Hamlyn B, Brooker S, Oleinkova K *et al.,* op. cit.

104 Renfrew MJ, Dyson L, Wallace L *et al.,* op. cit.

105 Porteous R, Kaufman K, Rush J. The effect of individualised professional support on the duration of breastfeeding: a randomised controlled trial. *J Hum Lact.* 2000; **16:** 3003–8.

106 Serafino-Cross P, Donovan P. Effectiveness of professional breastfeeding home support. *J Nutr Educ.* 1992; **24:** 117–22.

107 Pollard DL. The effect of self-regulation on breastfeeding duration in primiparous mothers. *Dissertation Abstracts Int.* 1998; **59:** 4731.

108 Dennis C, Hodnett E, Gallop R *et al.,* op. cit.

109 Porteous R, Kaufman K, Rush J, op. cit.

110 Bliss MC, Wiklie J, Acredolo C *et al.* The effect of discharge pack formula and breast pumps on breastfeeding duration and choice of infant feeding method. *Birth.* 1997; **24:** 90–107.

111 Renfrew MJ, Woolridge MW, Ross McGill H, op. cit.

112 Ibid.

113 Ibid.

114 Ibid.

115 Renfrew MJ, Dyson L, Wallace L *et al.*, op. cit.

116 Hauck YI, Dimmock JE. Evaluation of an information booklet on breastfeeding duration: a clinical trial. *J Adv Nurs.* 1994; **20**: 836–43.

117 Gunn J, Lumley J, Chondros P *et al.* Does an early check-up improve maternal health? Results from a randomised trial in Australian general practice. *Br J Obstet Gynaecol.* 1998; **105**: 991–7.

118 Gagnon AJ, Dougherty G, Jimenez V *et al.* Randomized trial of postpartum care after hospital discharge. *Pediatrics.* 2002; **109**: 80.

119 Renfrew MJ, Woolridge MW, Ross McGill H, op. cit.

120 Coombs DW, Reynolds K, Joyner G *et al.* A self-help program to increase breastfeeding among low-income women. *J Nutr Educ.* 1998; **30**: 203–9.

121 Serwint JR, Wilson ME, Vogelhut JW *et al.* A randomized controlled trial of prenatal pediatric visits for urban, low-income families. *Pediatrics.* 1996; **98**: 1069–75.

122 Howard C, Howard F, Lawrence R *et al.* Office prenatal formula advertising and its effect on breastfeeding patterns. *Obstet Gynecol.* 2000; **95**: 296–303.

CHAPTER 5

Breastfeeding and nutrition

Despite variations, breast milk will provide sufficient energy and protein to meet requirements for most infants during the first six months of life.

INTRODUCTION

This chapter identifies and discusses the nutritional benefits to the infant of breast milk, as well as the nutritional implications for the mother of breast-feeding her baby. This will enable the professional to be proactive in providing women with targeted information and discussing the nutritional aspects of breastfeeding.

As well as having an essential nutritional role, breast milk has a number of protective prebiotic functions and a number of bioactive components.[1] The composition of human milk varies widely among women, and can be influenced by such factors as biochemical individuality, maternal nutrition, and stage of gestation and lactation within the same woman.[2] Composition can also vary from day to day, from breast to breast, and within a feed (i.e. the difference between fore- and hind-milk).[3] Nevertheless, despite this wide inter-individual variation in breast milk composition, the breast milk of most women will provide sufficient energy and protein to meet the requirements of most infants during the first 6 months of life.[4]

Table 5.1 shows the composition of both human and cow's milk, and it can be used as a reference point throughout this chapter.

INFANT NUTRITION AND BREASTFEEDING

In this section, detailed information is provided on the various constituents of breast milk as they relate to the growth and development of the infant.

TABLE 5.1: Constituents of human and cow's milk (table reproduced with permission of the *Food and Nutrition Bulletin*[5])

Contents	Human milk	Cow's milk
Fat		
Total (g/100 ml)	4.2	3.8
Fatty acids ≤ 8C (%)	Trace	6
Polyunsaturated fatty acids (%)	14	3
Protein (g/100 ml)		
Total	1.1	3.3
Casein 0.4	0.3	2.5
α-Lactalbumin	0.3	0.1
Lactoferrin	0.2	Trace
IgA	0.1	0.003
IgG	0.001	0.06
Lysozyme	0.05	Trace
Serum albumin	0.05	0.03
β-Lactoglobulin	–	0.3
Carbohydrate (g/100 ml)		
Lactose	7.0	4.8
Oligosaccharides	0.5	0.005
Minerals (g/100 ml)		
Calcium	0.030	0.125
Phosphorus	0.014	0.093
Sodium	0.015	0.047
Potassium	0.055	0.155
Chlorine	0.043	0.103

Energy

Breast milk contains approximately 280 kJ (67 kcal) per 100 ml, with approximately 50% of its energy derived from fat, 40% from carbohydrate and the remaining 10% from protein. Variation between women in the energy content of breast milk is mainly due to differences in fat content.[6]

Protein

The protein content of mature breast milk is approximately 8–13 g/l and, like the content of other nutrients, it changes according to the stage of lactation. The protein content of colostrum is approximately 20 g/l,[7] much higher than that of mature milk. At about 2 weeks postpartum, breast milk contains 12.7 g/l, and it then declines gradually until it reaches a plateau at about 8 g/l by the fourth month, where it remains relatively stable until it falls substantially once weaning is well advanced.[8]

The protein content of breast milk is less than a third of that of cow's milk, which means that breast milk has a much lower renal solute load than unmodified cow's milk. Furthermore, about two-thirds of the protein is whey, which is much easier for the baby to digest than casein, whereas cow's milk contains mainly casein and only 20% whey.

The main proteins in the whey fraction of breast milk are α-lactalbumin and lactoferrin, which provide a complete source of essential amino acids, including taurine, which is present in high concentrations in human milk, but is absent from cow's milk.

A more detailed comparison of the protein content of breast and cow's milk is provided in Table 5.1.

Taurine

Whereas adults can synthesise taurine from other amino acids, infants have a limited ability to synthesise taurine, which is therefore an essential amino acid that must be provided in the diet. High concentrations of taurine are found in parts of the central nervous system, and it is thought to be important for the development of the central nervous system and the eye.[9]

Immunoprotective proteins

Breast milk also contains significant amounts of immunoprotective proteins such as secretory immunoglobulin A (IgA), lactoferrin and lysozyme, which play a role in protecting infants from gastrointestinal and respiratory infections. It is rare for an infant to be allergic to its mother's milk, whereas the main protein in cow's milk is β-lactalbumin, which may evoke an allergic response in some infants.

Fat

Variations have been found in the fat content of milk from women living in affluent and developing countries. Among pooled studies of women from affluent populations, the mean fat content was 4.3% at 30 days, and 4.6% at 90 days postpartum. However, the mean fat content of the milk of women in developing countries was significantly lower, being 3.5% at 30 days and 3.1% at 90 days postpartum. It has been observed that the fat content of breast milk is proportional to the amount of body fat of the mother, which is assumed to be lower in undernourished women in developing countries. The difference between the percentage of fat in women from affluent populations and that in women from developing populations may affect the infant.

Jensen and colleagues identified a variety of factors which have a minor effect on total fat content.[10] Three of these relate to within-feed factors, between-feed factors and duration of breastfeeding.

1   There is wide 'within-feed' variation, with hind-milk having a higher fat content than fore-milk. Neville reported that the average lipid content of breast milk at the end of a feed was double that at the beginning of a feed.[11]
2   The length of time between breastfeeds has been shown to have a negative influence on fat content. That is, as the time interval between feeds increases, the fat content of the subsequent feed decreases.
3   The fat content of breast milk increases slightly as the infant ages, but decreases after the initiation of weaning.

Omega-6 and omega-3 long-chain polyunsaturated fatty acids (LC-PUFAs)

Most fatty acids can be synthesised in the body, but humans are unable to produce two types of fatty acids, namely linoleic acid (18:2 omega-6) and α-linolenic acid (18:3 omega-3). These are termed *essential fatty acids*, as they must be consumed in the diet. They are then converted into long-chain polyunsaturated fatty acids (LC-PUFA) – linoleic acid into arachidonic acid (ARA) and α-linolenic acid into docosahexaenoic acid (DHA).[12]

LC-PUFAs and brain function

These two long-chain polyunsaturated fatty acids play important structural and functional roles in the body, and it is thought that they are necessary for the development of normal brain and visual function. ARA and DHA are both major structural components of neural tissues, and DHA is also a component of retinal photoreceptor membranes.[13] As the production of ARA and DHA from linoleic acid and α-linolenic acid is rather inefficient, the infant must obtain these two LC-PUFAs directly from exogenous sources (i.e. from their diet).

Whereas breast milk contains ARA and DHA, most standard infant formulas contain little or no ARA and DHA. Infants who are fed unsupplemented formula have been shown to have lower levels of DHA and ARA in the plasma phospholipids and cerebral cortex compared with breastfed infants.[14]

Reports that breastfed infants have a higher IQ and perform better on developmental tests than formula-fed infants led to the hypothesis that this might be related to an inadequate intake of LC-PUFAs.[15] This hypothesis has been tested by numerous researchers, who have investigated the effects of supplementing infant formula with ARA and DHA in both preterm and healthy term infants. The results of these studies have been evaluated and summarised in several review papers.[16,17]

Although the findings are not consistent across all studies, there is reasonable evidence to suggest that preterm infants who receive formula supplemented with DHA have improved visual attention and cognitive performance compared with infants who receive no DHA. For term infants the findings are less consistent, with less than 50% of all studies finding beneficial effects of LC-PUFAs on visual, mental or psychomotor functions.[18]

At the time of writing, formula manufacturers are not required by law to add these LC-PUFAs to infant formulas. However, most manufacturers do add these components to at least one of their product ranges, often promoting it as a premium product compared with their standard unsupplemented product.

Carbohydrates
Lactose
Breast milk contains about 70 g/l of carbohydrate, most of which is lactose. As well as being an important source of energy, it may have a number of important physiological roles. A small amount of lactose (about 10%) survives absorption in the small intestine and is fermented in the large intestine by colonic bacteria to form short-chain fatty acids and lactate. These reduce the colonic pH, which aids the absorption of calcium. Lactose also promotes the growth of lactobacilli, and may help to develop a 'friendly' colonic flora that protects against gastrointestinal infection.[19]

Cow's milk contains less lactose than breast milk, and in the manufacture of infant formula additional carbohydrate needs to be added to bring the total sugar level up to that of breast milk. Although some manufacturers add lactose, other glucose polymers are often used. These alternative carbohydrate sources in formula do not have the non-nutritive functional properties of lactose.[20]

Oligosaccharides
Breast milk contains a complex mixture of approximately 130 oligosaccharides that are present in only minute amounts in the milk of other mammals. The biological function of oligosaccharides is not fully understood. Quantitatively they are one of the main components of breast milk, and are thought to play an important role in preventing infectious diseases in the newborn infant.[21]

Oligosaccharides are only partially digested in the small intestine, so they reach the colon, where they stimulate the growth of bifidobacteria and lactobacilli in the intestine. These bacteria are thought to be beneficial to human health, in particular by preventing or reducing the risk of gastrointestinal infection.[22]

In addition to promoting the growth of these intestinal 'friendly' bacteria, oligosaccharides appear to bind with various bacteria, such as E. coli and Helicobacter pylori. This prevents these and other pathogenic bacteria from attaching to the mucosal surface of the intestine and spreading.[23] Oligosaccharides may also be important as a source of sialic acid, which is essential for brain development.

Trials of formulas that contain galacto-fructo-oligosaccharides have shown that it is possible to mimic the prebiotic effect of breast milk oligosaccharides not only by increasing the bifidobacteria, but also by producing an intestinal flora that is more like that of breastfed infants.[24] However, the subsequent effect on infant health has been less well studied. Nevertheless, in recent years most formula manufacturers have added galacto- and/or fructo-oligosaccharides to one or all of their preparations in recognition of their potential importance to infant health.

Vitamins

In general, the vitamin and mineral content of breast milk is sufficient to meet the nutritional needs of a healthy, full-term infant for the first 6 months of life. Some of the key vitamins and minerals will now be discussed in more detail.

Vitamin A

The transfer of vitamin A from maternal blood to breast milk is regulated by the amount of vitamin A in the serum. Serum vitamin A levels are not only affected by a woman's intake of vitamin A, but can also be reduced if she has low zinc status, protein-energy malnutrition or infection. The mature breast milk of healthy, well-nourished women will contain approximately 700 mg/l of vitamin A, but for women in developing countries the level may be half this. The concentration of vitamin A decreases slightly across the duration of lactation. In populations where vitamin A deficiency is endemic, the content of human milk may be supplemented and can only be corrected through maternal and/or infant supplementation, or complementary feeding for infants.[25]

In the UK, the recommended intake of vitamin A for infants up to 12 months of age is 350 mg/day (approximately 1200 IU/day), which will be readily supplied by breast milk. However, in developing countries where maternal vitamin A deficiency is common, more than 50% of infants may have serum vitamin A levels indicative of subclinical vitamin A deficiency (< 0.7 mmol/l). Despite this, breastfeeding is promoted as the best way of preventing vitamin A deficiency, and the risk of developing xerophthalmia and mortality in deprived populations is lower in breastfed infants than in non-breastfed infants.[26]

Vitamin D

Rickets caused by vitamin D deficiency was commonly observed in children in industrialised cities in the UK and Europe until around the middle of the twentieth century, when milk was supplemented with vitamin D in most countries.[27] Case reports of infants presenting with clinical signs of rickets started to reappear in the medical literature in the 1990s. Almost all cases of rickets in the USA were African-American infants who had been breastfed without vitamin D supplementation.[28] It has been suggested that the reappearance of rickets in industrialised countries during the later decades of the twentieth century may be an unintended consequence of the promotion of breastfeeding.[29]

Among Western countries the recommended dietary intake of vitamin D for infants under 12 months of age ranges from 7.5 to 10 mg. The average range of vitamin D concentration in breast milk from healthy women who are not vitamin deficient is 10–60 IU/l (0.25–1.5 mg/l).[30] The vitamin D content of human milk is highly variable, and is directly related to maternal serum levels.

It has also been shown that the vitamin D content of the milk of dark-skinned women is lower than that of white-skinned women.[31]

There are relatively few dietary sources of vitamin D, and we obtain most of our daily vitamin D requirements from the synthesis of vitamin D_3 in the skin. Solar ultraviolet B radiation converts a pre-vitamin D in the skin into the active form, vitamin D_3.

The vitamin D content of breast milk is not sufficient to meet infant requirements, yet the incidence of rickets among breastfed infants is still very low, particularly in infants under 6 months of age. However, most breastfed infants receive adequate amounts of vitamin D through a combination of breast milk and casual exposure to sunlight.[32] It is estimated that exposure to sunlight for 30 minutes per week (nappy only) or 2 hours per week (fully clothed, no hat) will maintain adequate serum vitamin D levels.

Although nutritional rickets is uncommon in countries where sunlight is plentiful, it is a problem in countries at or above 40°N or below 40°S, where sunlight is limited for large parts of the year, and the cold weather results in people wearing layers of clothes that cover most of their body, thus limiting their exposure to natural sunlight. In northern countries, vitamin D levels in breast milk are lower in winter, when women have less exposure to sunlight.

It is thought that dark-skinned infants living in countries where sunlight is limited are at greater risk of vitamin D deficiency than Caucasian children, due to their increased skin pigmentation, which necessitates considerably longer exposure to sunlight. Nutritional rickets has been observed in Muslim families in the UK and the USA, and this is likely to be related to lack of exposure to sunlight for cultural reasons, exacerbated by increased skin pigmentation.[33] The parents of dark-skinned children and/or children with limited exposure to sunlight need to know about their infants' increased risk of vitamin D deficiency and the need for supplementation. It is the responsibility of the healthcare professional to be aware of such issues and to provide culturally specific advice on breastfeeding.

The re-emergence of vitamin D deficiency in vulnerable populations, coupled with concerns about the hazardous effects of exposure to ultraviolet light, led to the recommendation by the American Academy of Pediatrics that all full-term breastfed infants should receive at least 200 IU (5 mg) of vitamin D per day, beginning in the first 2 months after delivery.[34]

This recommendation is controversial because it does not apply to formula-fed infants, as infant formula is supplemented with vitamin D. Healthcare professionals are concerned that a blanket recommendation that all breastfed infants should be supplemented may imply that breast milk is somehow inadequate, and could undermine a mother's confidence in the adequacy of her breast milk, creating another barrier to the successful promotion of breastfeeding.[35]

However, it should be noted that in Canada a recommendation was introduced in the early 1990s that breastfed infants should be supplemented with 10 mg of vitamin D, and this has had no apparent adverse effects on breastfeeding, as rates have continued to rise since that time.[36]

Folate

Breast milk contains high levels of folate, and the folate content of breast milk is maintained at the expense of the mother's folate status.[37] Folate levels do not fall unless the mother is severely depleted, and this is unlikely to occur in women living in countries with mandatory folate fortification, or in women who follow health recommendations to take folic acid supplements during pregnancy and lactation.

Vitamin B_6

Vitamin B_6 deficiency in infancy is associated with compromised linear growth but not with compromised weight. The vitamin B_6 content of milk is dependent on maternal status and intake, and breast milk content will be suboptimal among women at risk of vitamin B_6 deficiency.

Minerals

Table 5.1 lists several minerals that are found in both breast and cow's milk. In this section, iron and zinc will be briefly discussed.

Iron

Although breast milk has a relatively low concentration of iron, the iron has a high bioavailability, with 50% or more being absorbed.[38] The iron requirements of an infant cannot be met by human milk alone, but the iron from milk is supplemented from the stores that the baby is born with.

Iron deficiency is therefore unlikely to occur in full-term, normal-birthweight infants who have been exclusively breastfed for around 6 months. However, preterm infants who are born with incomplete iron stores are vulnerable to iron deficiency during the first year of life.[39] Iron deficiency in early childhood is usually related to insufficient iron intake from a mixed solid food and milk diet. Continued breastfeeding into the second year of life helps to reduce the risk of deficiency once weaning has commenced.

Zinc

Like iron, the zinc in breast milk is highly bioavailable, which compensates for its low concentration. Although the absorption of zinc falls short of an infant's zinc requirements, it appears to be supplemented by prenatal stores,[40] and zinc deficiency is rare in exclusively breastfed infants before 6 months of age.[41]

Renal solute load

The protein and mineral content of breast milk contributes to its renal solute load, which is lower than that of cow's milk and normal infant formula. The ability of the kidney to handle a dietary solute load is reflected in plasma osmolality.[42] Breastfed infants have a lower mean plasma osmolality than formula-fed infants. The immature kidney is unable to excrete a high renal solute load, and this is one of the reasons for recommending that the introduction of unmodified cow's milk and solids to infants should be delayed.[43]

Protective and bioactive components of breast milk

As well as fulfilling an essential nutritional role, breast milk contains a number of non-nutritional components, including protective and bioactive components. Some of these non-nutritional components have already been identified and discussed. The roles of the main non-nutritional components of breast milk are summarised in Table 5.2.

MATERNAL NUTRITION AND BREASTFEEDING

This section provides detailed information on the effects of breastfeeding on maternal nutrition, and how maternal nutrition may affect the composition of

TABLE 5.2: Examples of the non-nutritional components of breast milk (table reproduced with permission of the *Food and Nutrition Bulletin*[44])

Antimicrobial factors	Growth factors
Secretory IgA, IgM, IgG	Epidermal (EGF)
Lactoferrin	Nerve (NGF)
Lysozyme	Insulin-like (IGF)
Complement C3	Transforming (TGF)
Leucocytes	Taurine
Bifidus factor	Polyamines
Lipids and fatty acids	
Antiviral mucins, GAGs	
Oligosaccharides	

Cytokines and anti-inflammatory factors	Digestive enzymes
Tumour necrosis factor	Amylase
Interleukins	Bile-acid-stimulating esterase
Interferon-γ	Bile-acid-stimulating lipases
Prostaglandins	Lipoprotein lipase
α_1-Antichymotrypsin	
α_1-Antitrypsin	
Platelet-activating factor: acetyl hydrolase	

(*continued*)

TABLE 5.2: (*continued*)

Hormones	Transporters
Feedback inhibitor of lactation (FIL)	Lactoferrin (Fe)
Insulin	Folate binder
Prolactin	Cobalamin binder
Thyroid hormones	IgF binder
Corticosteroids, ACTH	Thyroxine binder
Oxytocin	Corticosteroid binder
Calcitonin	
Parathyroid hormone	
Erythropoietin	

Potentially harmful substances	Others
Viruses (e.g. HIV)	Casomorphins
Aflatoxins	δ-Sleep peptides
Trans-fatty acids	Nucleotides
Nicotine, caffeine	DNA, RNA
Food allergens	
PCBs, DDT, dioxins	
Radioisotopes	
Drugs	

breast milk. An initial starting point is evidence that, with some exceptions, the nutrient intake of the mother appears to have only a slight effect on milk volume, or on transfer of nutrients to the baby.[45] Therefore it can be assumed that in women who are well nourished, milk production will not be affected to any great extent by maternal diet. Importantly, however, milk production will fall following the introduction of formula feeding and/or complementary foods, as has already been discussed in previous chapters.

Milk volume

Physiologically, the volume of milk produced by women is relatively consistent across population groups, regardless of their nutritional status.[46] So long as they are not starving, it appears that most women are able to produce at least 700 ml of breast milk per day. As has already been discussed in previous chapters, infant demand is the main mechanism for regulating milk volume, and the latter is also influenced by the weight of the infant.[47]

The energy needs of lactating women

The main factors that influence the energy needs of lactating women are the duration of breastfeeding and the extent of exclusive breastfeeding.[48] During the third trimester of pregnancy, most well-nourished women lay down fat stores which are intended to be mobilised to subsidise the cost of lactation during the first few months of breastfeeding.[49] Postpartum weight loss is usually highest in the first 3 months, and women who exclusively breastfeed tend to lose more weight than those who partially breastfeed.

On average, lactating women lose about 0.2–0.8 kg/month during the first 6 months postpartum, but weight loss is slower (around 0.1–0.2 kg/month) during the second 6 months.[50]

The extent to which mobilised fat stores offset the energy costs of lactation depends on the amount of weight that a woman gains during pregnancy and/or her nutritional status.[51]

The Food and Agriculture Organization (FAO) recommends that well-nourished women with adequate gestational weight gain should increase their food intake by 2.1 MJ/day (500 kcal/day) for the first 6 months of lactation, whereas undernourished women and those with insufficient gestational weight gain should increase their food intake by 2.8 MJ/day (675 kcal/day).[52] The energy requirements will be lower for women who partially breastfeed. Energy requirements decrease after 6 months to an additional 1.7 MJ/day (400 kcal/day).

The energy cost of lactation can be determined by calculating the product of breast milk volume, milk energy density, and the efficiency of conversion of dietary energy to breast milk energy. The total energy requirement for lactating women is then derived by adding this product to the energy needs of non-pregnant, non-lactating (NPNL) women, with adjustments being made for changes in physical activity and changes in body fat.[53] Figure 5.1 demonstrates this method.

Energy reserves

Evidence from both human and animal studies indicates that, regardless of energy balance, milk volume and milk energy output will be maintained within the expected ranges in females with adequate energy reserves, and also in females with low energy reserves who are not losing weight.[54] It is only when a woman has low energy reserves and also an inadequate energy intake that milk energy output is predicted to decrease. In developing countries where chronic undernutrition is common, some researchers have reported an association between postpartum weight loss and lower milk energy transfer.[55] A review paper by Lederman describes the influence of lactation on body weight regulation.[56]

Breast milk volume x milk energy density × conversion efficiency
+
NPNL energy requirements (± changes in physical activity)
±
changes in body fat

FIGURE 5.1: Calculation of maternal energy requirements during lactation.

The evidence from studies in both Western and developing societies suggests that during the early stages of lactation, women meet the increased energy demands of lactation primarily by increasing their intake of energy and reducing their level of physical activity.

The promotion and support of breastfeeding beyond 6 months may help women to lose body fat during the postpartum period. This may be important in helping to decrease the development of obesity among women of reproductive age, particularly in Western countries, where excessive weight gain during pregnancy is relatively common.

Protein

The additional protein that is required during lactation is calculated by estimating the amount of dietary protein needed to support production of a given amount of protein in milk.[57] The amount of protein will depend on the total volume of breast milk produced, which is in turn influenced by the age of the infant and whether the mother is exclusively or partially breastfeeding. The additional levels of protein recommended by the FAO, the WHO and the United Nations University (UNU) are as follows:

➤ 16–17 g/day for 0–6 months of lactation
➤ 12.3 g/day for 6–12 months of lactation
➤ 11.3 g/day for 12–24 months of lactation.

In developed countries, the protein intake typically exceeds the requirements of NPNL women, so the protein costs of lactation are easily met, and most women do not need to make a special effort to increase the protein sources in their diet. A low protein intake is unlikely to affect milk volume, but there is mixed evidence to suggest that the concentration of certain fractions of milk protein may be altered.[58]

Fat

The total fat content of breast milk does not appear to be significantly affected by how much fat a woman eats. However, the quality of fat (i.e. the fatty acid profile) is influenced by her diet. The LC-PUFA content of breast milk is influenced by a woman's diet, and the content of DHA in particular is highly variable. There will be cultural variations in fat content that reflect prevailing dietary habits.

As infants cannot synthesise the essential fatty acid precursors of ARA and DHA, lactating women need to ensure that their diet contains sources of these LC-PUFAs. The primary dietary sources of the latter are egg yolk (ARA and DHA), oily fish (mainly DHA) and red meat. Vegetable oils are rich sources of the precursor essential fatty acids – linoleic acid is found in sunflower and maize oils, and α-linolenic acid is found in soybean and rapeseed oils. Finley *et al.* have reported that the breast milk of vegetarian women contains a lower concentration of essential fatty acids derived from animal sources and a higher concentration of polyunsaturated fatty acids derived from vegetable sources.[59]

It has also been reported that the breast milk of Spanish women contains higher levels of linoleic acid than have been reported for other groups of women, due to a high proportion of polyunsaturated fat intake from vegetable oils.[60]

The ARA content of breast milk is less variable, and is not as readily influenced by the maternal diet.[61] The milk of vegetarian women contains less DHA than that of women who eat meat, while the DHA content in milk of women with a high fish intake is higher than that of women who rarely or never eat fish.[62] Studies have shown that the concentration of DHA in human milk can be increased by the use of supplements containing DHA,[63] or through the increased consumption of oily fish, such as herring and mackerel. Lactating women should be encouraged to consume two servings of fish per week, particularly oil-rich fish such as mackerel, herring and sardines.

Vitamins and minerals

The vitamin content of human milk is affected by a number of factors, of which the nutritional status of the mother is the most important. In general, when maternal vitamin intake is low, human milk levels are reduced and respond to supplementation, whereas when maternal vitamin intake is high, milk vitamin levels approach a plateau and are less responsive to supplementation.[64] It is rare for exclusively breastfed infants of undernourished women to demonstrate clinical signs of micronutrient deficiencies.[65]

Milk concentrations of iron, zinc and calcium are not reduced when the mother is deficient, so she is vulnerable to further depletion during lactation.[66] With the notable exception of zinc, maternal intake and deficiency of minerals therefore generally do not affect the mineral content of breast milk.

Vitamin A

In general, breast milk is a rich source of vitamin A and, even in deprived populations, vitamin A deficiency in infancy is relatively rare.[67] The breast milk of well-nourished women will contain adequate vitamin A. However, in countries with endemic vitamin A deficiency, the vitamin A concentration of breast milk can be low, and infants may become depleted. High-dose supplements of vitamin A can improve the mother's vitamin A stores and breast milk vitamin A levels.[68]

Vitamin D

There are relatively few dietary sources of vitamin D. Oily fish, liver and egg yolks provide modest amounts, with additional small amounts being obtained from fortified foods such as milk, margarine and breakfast cereals in some countries. Studies have shown that maternal supplementation with vitamin D can increase breast milk levels of this vitamin, as can exposure to UV light.[69] Although the available data indicate that vitamin D requirements are not increased during lactation, a supplement of vitamin D (10 mg/day) is recommended for vegetarian women and those who avoid milk and other foods fortified with vitamin D.[70]

Vitamin D supplementation is especially important for those women who have limited exposure to sunlight and/or who have dark skin, as discussed earlier in this chapter.

Vitamin B$_{12}$

Women who are ovo-lacto vegetarians or who consume small amounts of meat are at greater risk of vitamin B$_{12}$ deficiency than are omnivores. Vitamin B$_{12}$ deficiency has been reported in the breastfed offspring of vegetarian women. These groups of women, but in particular lactating women who consume a vegan diet, should be encouraged to take a vitamin B$_{12}$ supplement.[71]

Infants of breastfeeding women with untreated pernicious anaemia may on occasion experience vitamin B$_{12}$ deficiency. In these circumstances the lactating mother should be given parenteral vitamin B$_{12}$ to treat the pernicious anaemia and increase the vitamin B$_{12}$ level of her milk.

Iron

An interesting research finding is that a relatively large proportion of women are anaemic at the start of their pregnancy.[72] The recommended intake of iron for a lactating woman is about half that recommended for an NPNL woman. This is calculated on the assumption that menstruation does not resume until around 6 months postpartum, and hence the need to replace menstrual iron losses is reduced.

However, research evidence has drawn attention to the fact that a relatively large proportion of women, especially those in developing countries and women on a low income in Western countries, enter pregnancy with anaemia or low iron stores, and subsequently have a high risk of postpartum anaemia.[73,74] For instance, a high prevalence of postpartum anaemia has been reported among women on a low income in the USA, where the prevalence was 27% overall, and 48% among black American women.[75]

Picciano has suggested that the recommended iron intake during lactation should be increased to allow for the recovery of iron stores and the possibility of postpartum iron-deficiency anaemia.[76] The iron content of breast milk does not appear to be influenced by maternal diet, but supplementation is important for the health of iron-deficient lactating women.

Calcium

Frank calcium deficiency is rare in breastfed infants. Breast milk contains 250–300 mg/l of calcium, and the concentration does not change substantially during lactation. The concentration of calcium in milk does not appear to be influenced by maternal diet, with breast milk levels being maintained at the expense of maternal bone demineralisation among women with low calcium intake. However, there is some evidence that women with a habitually low intake of calcium produce milk with lower than normal calcium levels.[77]

In their review paper, Emmett and Rogers describe the properties of human milk and whether or not they are affected by maternal diet, and Butte *et al*. have evaluated the nutritional adequacy of exclusive breastfeeding in a comprehensive review prepared for the World Health Organization.[78,79] These are useful texts to consult for further information on this topic.

OTHER SUBSTANCES TRANSFERRED IN BREAST MILK
Flavours
Flavours such as garlic, mint, vanilla and alcohol are volatile compounds and can be absorbed by milk, thus changing its taste. This has potential benefits when it comes to introducing solid foods, as human and animal studies have shown that offspring show a preference for foods to which they have been exposed from their mother's diet during pregnancy and lactation.[80] For instance, in one study breastfed infants ate significantly more of a new vegetable than formula-fed infants when they were exposed to it for the first time.[81] Breast milk appears to provide the infant with a variety of chemosensory experiences, and may facilitate their acceptance of new foods at the time of weaning and lay the foundation for future food preferences.

Alcohol
Traditionally in many societies alcohol has been promoted to stimulate the production of breast milk. There is no scientific evidence to support this claim, and mothers and healthcare professionals should be aware that moderate amounts of alcohol may decrease breast milk production and may also have a detrimental effect on motor development.[82] Despite the lack of scientific evidence, women were often advised to take alcoholic beverages such as beer and stout to improve both the quality and quantity of their milk.

Recent research indicates that rather than being a 'galactogenic' substance, alcohol when consumed in moderate quantities (0.4 g/kg body weight, equivalent to two or three standard drinks) in fact decreases oxytocin levels and consequently the volume of milk produced.[83]

Alcohol is transferred to the infant via breast milk, but the amount is likely to be low if a mother's alcohol intake is moderate (i.e. no more than one or two standard drinks per day). Limited research in animals and infants indicates that alcohol ingested via breast milk may have a slight adverse effect on motor development.[84] Although the consumption of alcohol does not preclude a woman from breastfeeding, lactating women should be advised to drink alcohol in small amounts, if at all.

Environmental smoke
Studies have shown that infants who are exposed to environmental smoke have a higher risk of developing respiratory infections than infants who live in non-smoking households. However, it appears that breastfeeding offers protection to infants who are exposed to environmental smoke. In a Norwegian study, infants

of mothers who smoked and who had breastfed for less than 6 months had twice the risk of lower respiratory tract infections (LRTI) compared with infants of non-smoking mothers who had breastfed for 6 months or more. However, breastfed infants of smokers who breastfed for more than 6 months had a risk of LRTI similar to that of infants of non-smokers who breastfed for more than 6 months.[85]

A general rule is that lactating women should be encouraged to stop smoking, and supported in doing so, for the benefit of their own health and that of their baby.

Numerous studies in various countries have shown a negative association between smoking and breastfeeding duration. However, as women who smoke are less likely to intend to breastfeed, it is unlikely that smoking has a physiological effect on breastfeeding duration. It is more likely that the lower rates of breastfeeding among women who smoke are related to psychological factors, in so far as women who smoke have less motivation to breastfeed.[86]

Heavy metals

Heavy metals such as lead and mercury have been shown to adversely affect brain development in young children. Unless a woman has been accidentally exposed to high levels during pregnancy and lactation, these heavy metals are only detected in breast milk at trace levels, which are unlikely to cause harm to the breastfed infant. Nevertheless, where applicable, women should be advised of the theoretical risk associated with these heavy metals through exposure to lead-based paints (now banned in most countries, but which may have been used in older buildings and toys) and to fish from certain areas contaminated with heavy metals, such as mercury and cadmium.

Other environmental contaminants

Many industrial processes produce unwanted by-products known as persistent organic pollutants (POP). These include vinyl and polyvinyl chloride (PVC) plastic manufacturing, medical waste, garbage and hazardous waste incineration, home, building and vehicle fires, and pesticides. These pollutants are resistant to degradation, and so spread through the water, soil and air and are ingested and stored by fish and animals, eventually reaching us through the food chain.[87] Once ingested, POPS are stored in fat tissue, and they are unlikely to be excreted except through breast milk.[88]

Detectable levels of a number of organochlorine pesticides (e.g. DDT) and polychlorinated biphenyls (PCBs) have been found in the breast milk of women, even in those countries where the use of these compounds has been banned for 20 years or more. In developing countries where these pesticides and chemicals are still in use, the levels of these contaminants in breast milk remain high.[89] Levels of POP in breast milk tend to be higher in first-time mothers, and also tend to be higher during the first months of breastfeeding.[90]

It is difficult to estimate the health risks associated with the levels of POP currently found in breast milk. In countries where the use of these compounds is banned the risks are low, and even in countries where they are still in use the risks are outweighed by the benefits of breastfeeding. Although formulas contain less POP than human milk, there are still risks to the formula-fed infant via water contaminated with chemicals, and potential contaminants in teats and bottles and in the formula itself. In addition there are, as discussed in previous chapters, well-documented risks of infection associated with formula feeding. Even in countries where there may be exposure to environmental chemicals, the hazards associated with contaminated breast milk can be considered to be less than the hazards associated with formula feeding.

There are a number of contaminants that may be transferred to the infant via the mother's milk. Some of the more common ones have been reviewed briefly, but a more detailed description can be found in a review by Golding.[91] The National Resources Defense Council website (www.nrdc.org/breastmilk/chems. asp) also includes an informative discussion about chemical contaminants in breast milk and the health risks associated with POP.

ANTIGEN AVOIDANCE

There is limited evidence from randomised controlled trials to suggest that if a high-risk woman adopts an antigen-avoidance diet during lactation, she may substantially reduce the likelihood of her child developing atopic eczema. However, there is no evidence at this stage that an antigen-avoidance diet in mothers will improve the symptoms of infants with existing atopic eczema.[92]

It may be advisable for women with a personal history of atopic allergy, or with one or more previous children with atopic eczema, to avoid hyperallergenic foods such as cow's milk and eggs while breastfeeding. However, the potential benefits of reducing the risk of allergy in the infant need to be balanced against the potential risk of the mother consuming a nutritionally unbalanced diet. Women should receive guidance on suitable foods to substitute for milk and eggs in their diet.

CONCLUSION

Breast milk provides essential nutrition for the human infant, and has protective prebiotic functions and bioactive components. Whereas the volume of milk produced is relatively consistent across population groups with a wide range of nutritional conditions, the composition of breast milk varies widely among women and at various times of breastfeeding in direct relationship with individual factors. Despite variations, breast milk will provide sufficient energy and protein to meet the requirements of most infants during the first 6 months of life. In well-nourished women, milk production is not affected to any great extent by maternal diet, but milk production will fall following the introduction of formula feeding and/or complementary foods.

Healthcare professionals need to understand fully the nutritional implications of breastfeeding for the mother and the infant. This chapter therefore demonstrates the considerable advantages to both mother and baby of breastfeeding, and has identified the issues that healthcare professionals may encounter and be required to address in the course of their work.

FURTHER READING

The Centers for Disease Control and Prevention (CDC) have published a report of the Vitamin D Expert Panel meeting, which is useful for healthcare professionals who wish to review the evidence about the need for a blanket recommendation that all breastfed infants receive vitamin D supplementation. This can be accessed via their website (www.cdc.gov/nccdphp/dnpa/nutrition/pdf/vitamin_d_expert_panel_meeting.pdf).

The National Resources Defense Council provides information on chemical contamination and breast milk for a range of chemicals. Again this can be accessed via their website (www.nrdc.org/breastmilk/chems.asp).

In the UK, the National Institute for Health and Clinical Excellence (NICE) has produced and formally launched public health guidance entitled *Guidance for Midwives, Health Visitors, Pharmacists and Other Primary Care Services to Improve the Nutrition of Pregnant and Breastfeeding Mothers and Children in Low-Income Households* (available online at www.nice.org.uk/PH011). This document aims to address disparities in the nutrition of low-income and other disadvantaged groups compared with the general UK population, and specifically identifies breastfeeding promotion as an objective.

ACKNOWLEDGEMENT

We would like to gratefully acknowledge the contribution of Dr Jane Scott to the information about breastfeeding and nutrition.

REFERENCES

1 Michaelsen K, Weaver L, Branca F *et al*. *Feeding and Nutrition of Infants and Young Children. Guidelines for the WHO European region, with emphasis on the former Soviet countries*. Geneva: WHO Regional Publications; 2000.
2 Picciano M. Human milk: nutritional aspects of a dynamic food. *Biol Neonate*. 1998; **74**: 84–93.
3 Neville M. Studies on human lactation. I. Within-feed and between-breast variation in selected components of human milk. *Am J Clin Nutr*. 1984; **40**: 635–46.
4 Butte N, Lopez-Alarcon M, Garza C. *Nutrient Adequacy of Exclusive Breastfeeding for the Term Infant during the First Six Months of Life*. Geneva: World Health Organization; 2002.

5 Prentice A. Constituents of human milk. *Food Nutr Bull.* 1996; **17**. www.unu.edu/unupress/food/8F174e/8F174E00.htm (accessed 24 June 2010).

6 Emmett P, Rogers I. Properties of human milk and their relationship with maternal nutrition. *Early Hum Dev.* 1997; **49**: 7–28.

7 Ibid.

8 Butte N, Lopez-Alarcon M, Garza C, op. cit.

9 Emmett P, Rogers I, op. cit.

10 Jensen R, Ferris A, Lammi-Keefe C. Lipids in human milk and infant formulas. *Annu Rev Nutr.* 1992; **12**: 417–41.

11 Neville M, op. cit.

12 Forsyth S, Hornstra G. Essential fatty acids: maternal and infant nutrition. *Pract Midwife.* 2001; **4**: 34–7.

13 Heird W, Lapillonne A. The role of essential fatty acids in development. *Annu Rev Nutr.* 2005; **25**: 549–71.

14 Forsyth S, Hornstra G, op. cit.

15 Heird W, Lapillonne A, op. cit.

16 Fleith M, Clandinin M. Dietary PUFA for preterm and term infants: review of clinical studies. *Crit Rev Food Sci Nutr.* 2005; **45**: 205–29.

17 McCann J, Ames B. Is docosahexaenoic acid, an n-3 long-chain polyunsaturated fatty acid, required for development of normal brain function? An overview of evidence from cognitive and behavioural tests in humans and animals. *Am J Clin Nutr.* 2005; **82**: 281–95.

18 Fleith M, Clandinin M, op. cit.

19 Michaelsen K, Weaver L, Branca F *et al.*, op. cit.

20 Emmett P, Rogers I, op. cit.

21 Coppa G, Bruni S, Morelli L *et al.* The first prebiotics in humans: human milk oligo-saccharides. *J Clin Gastroenterol.* 2004; **38**: 80–83.

22 Bezkorovainy B. Probiotics: determinants of survival and growth in the gut. *Am J Clin Nutr.* 2001; **73**: 399–405.

23 Kunz C, Rudloff S, Baier W *et al.* Oligosaccharides in human milk: structural, functional and metabolic aspects. *Annu Rev Nutr.* 2000; **20**: 699–722.

24 Fanaro S, Boehm G, Garssen J *et al.* Galacto-oligosaccharides and long-chain fructo-oligosaccharides as prebiotics in infant formula: a review. *Acta Paediatr.* 2005; **94**: 22–6.

25 Butte N, Lopez-Alarcon M, Garza C, op. cit.

26 Bates C, Prentice A. Breast milk as a source of vitamins, essential minerals and trace elements. *Pharmacol Ther.* 1994; **62**: 193–220.

27 Henderson A. Vitamin D and the breastfed infant. *J Obstet Gynecol Neonatal Nurs.* 2005; **34**: 367–72.

28 Scanlon K. *Vitamin D Expert Panel Meeting: final report.* Atlanta, GA: Centers for Disease Control and Prevention; 2001.

29 Welch T. Vitamin D-deficient rickets: the re-emergence of a once-conquered disease. *J Pediatr.* 2000; **137**: 143–5.

30 Henderson A, op. cit.

31 Bates C, Prentice A, op. cit.

32 Henderson A, op. cit.

33 Scanlon K, op. cit.

34 Gartner LM, Greer FR, Section on Breastfeeding and Committee on Nutrition, American Academy of Pediatrics. Prevention of rickets and vitamin D deficiency: new guidelines for vitamin D intake. *Pediatrics.* 2003; **111**: 908–10.

35 Henderson A, op. cit.

36 Scanlon K, op. cit.

37 Emmett P, Rogers I, op. cit.

38 Department of Health. *Weaning and the Weaning Diet. Report of the Working Group on the Weaning Diet of the Committee on Medical Aspects of Food Policy.* London: HMSO; 1994.

39 Ibid.

40 Butte N, Lopez-Alarcon M, Garza C, op. cit.

41 Michaelsen K, Weaver L, Branca F *et al.*, op. cit.

42 Emmett P, Rogers I, op. cit.

43 Department of Health, op. cit.

44 Prentice A, op. cit.

45 Picciano M, op. cit.

46 Prentice A, Spaaij C, Goldberg G *et al.* Energy requirements of pregnant and lactating women. *Eur J Clin Nutr.* 1996; **50**: 82–111.

47 Emmett P, Rogers I, op. cit.

48 Food and Agriculture Organization. *Human Energy Requirements. Report of a Joint FAO/WHO/UNU Expert Consultation.* Rome: Food and Agriculture Organization; 2004.

49 Picciano M, op. cit.

50 Lederman S. Influence of lactation on body weight regulation. *Nutr Rev.* 2004; **62**: 112–19.

51 Food and Agriculture Organization, op. cit.

52 Ibid.

53 Dewey K. Energy and protein requirements during lactation. *Annu Rev Nutr.* 1997; **17**: 18–36.

54 Ibid.

55 Ibid.

56 Lederman S, op. cit.

57 Dewey K, op. cit.

58 Ibid.

59 Finley D, Lönnerdal B, Dewey K *et al.* Breast milk composition: fat content and fatty acid composition in vegetarians and non-vegetarians. *Am J Clin Nutr.* 1985; **41**: 787–800.

60 Barbas C, Herrera E. Lipid composition and vitamin E content in human colostrum and mature milk. *J Physiol Biochem.* 1998; **54**: 167–74.

61 Heird W, Lapillonne A, op. cit.

62 Finley D, Lönnerdal B, Dewey K *et al.*, op. cit.

63 Jensen R, Ferris A, Lammi-Keefe C, op. cit.

64 Picciano M, op. cit.

65 Michaelsen K, Weaver L, Branca F *et al.*, op. cit.

66 Ibid.

67 Allen L. Multiple micronutrients in pregnancy and lactation: an overview. *Am J Clin Nutr.* 2005; **81**: 1206–12.

68 Bates C, Prentice A, op. cit.

69 Ibid.

70 Picciano M, op. cit.

71 Ibid.

72 Ibid.

73 Ibid.

74 Allen L, op. cit.

75 Bodnar L, Scanlon K, Freedman D *et al.* High prevalence of postpartum anemia among low-income women in the United States. *Am J Obstet Gynecol.* 2001; **185:** 438–43.

76 Picciano M, op. cit.

77 Bates C, Prentice A, op. cit.

78 Emmett P, Rogers I, op. cit.

79 Butte N, Lopez-Alarcon M, Garza C, op. cit.

80 Mennella J, Jagnow C, Beauchamp G. Prenatal and postnatal flavor learning by human infants. *Pediatrics.* 2001; **107:** 88.

81 Sullivan S, Birch L. Infant dietary experience and acceptance of solid foods. *Pediatrics.* 1994; **93:** 271–7.

82 Golding J. Unnatural constituents of breast milk – medication, lifestyle, pollutants, viruses. *Early Hum Dev.* 1997; **49:** 29–43.

83 Mennella J, Jagnow C, Beauchamp G, op. cit.

84 Golding J, op. cit.

85 Nafstad P, Jaakola J, Hagen J *et al.* Breastfeeding, maternal smoking and lower respiratory tract infections. *Eur Respir J.* 1996; **9:** 2623–9.

86 Amir LH, Donath SM. Does maternal smoking have a negative physiological effect on breastfeeding? The epidemiological evidence. *Birth.* 2002; **29:** 112–23.

87 Natural Resources Defense Council. *Healthy Milk, Healthy Baby: chemical pollution and mother's milk.* www.nrdc.org/breastmilk/chems.asp (accessed 2 November 2009).

88 Golding J, op. cit.

89 Natural Resources Defense Council, op. cit.

90 Ibid.

91 Golding J, op. cit.

92 Kramer MS, Kakuma R. Maternal dietary antigen avoidance during pregnancy or lactation, or both, for preventing or treating atopic disease in the child. *Cochrane Database Syst Rev.* 2006; **3:** CD000133.

93 Butte N, Lopez-Alarcon M, Garza C, op. cit.

CHAPTER 6

Towards evidence-based practice

The Nursing and Midwifery Council (NMC), in its *Code: standards of conduct, performance and ethics for nurses and midwives*, stipulates that nurses and midwives should make use of the best evidence they are able to access.[1]

INTRODUCTION

The previous chapters provide clear evidence of the benefits of breastfeeding to mother and baby. A major challenge in contemporary times is that of 'information overload.' Women who are considering breastfeeding, as well the healthcare professionals who are aiming to promote and support breastfeeding, may find themselves having to consider a large volume of information. Helping women to untangle the mass of available information on breastfeeding is a major responsibility of the healthcare professional. Furthermore, demonstrating that practice is evidence based is a key aspect of the role of the healthcare professional in providing information and facilitating informed decision making by women that is based on their individual needs and circumstances.

This chapter is based on the belief that healthcare professionals play an essential role in promoting and initiating breastfeeding, as well as in helping mothers to continue breastfeeding. It also proposes that understanding and applying the available evidence will lead to best practice among healthcare professionals in breastfeeding promotion, initiation and continuation. It can also help interested professionals to be proactive in policy making and standards development at local, national and even international levels.

The chapter opens with an overview of what evidence-based practice is and the key components involved. Following on from this, evidence in five areas of research that are relevant to breastfeeding is examined, to demonstrate the increasingly essential part that research evidence is playing in the role of the healthcare professional. The research topics chosen are used to examine some of the issues and challenges underpinning evidence-based practice. Collectively these studies demonstrate how research has the potential to influence attitudes to breastfeeding either negatively or positively. They also show the necessity for healthcare professionals to have knowledge and competence in skills of critiquing and interpreting research studies and in using and transferring research evidence to develop professional practice and enhance the quality of healthcare services that are delivered to patients and clients.

The chapter concludes with a practice focus that describes the research process and includes information on research critique frameworks, which can help to guide healthcare professionals when appraising research articles.

IN SUPPORT OF EVIDENCE-BASED PRACTICE

Many different definitions of evidence-based practice have been put forward, but it is commonly accepted that, in healthcare, evidence-based practice aims to provide patient or client care which is based on the best available evidence. This includes evidence from research studies, but it may also include other forms of evidence, such as expert knowledge, clinical experience or local audit, as well as the preferences and needs of the patient.[2] For the professional whose work involves promoting and supporting breastfeeding, evidence-based practice will also include the ability to communicate and explain evidence to women in their care. Although the focus of this chapter is on the use of research evidence, it is important for healthcare professionals to contextualise their use of such evidence, by also considering the other types of evidence that are available to them, including their own clinical judgement and the needs of mothers and babies.

Evidence-based practice has its roots in medicine and specifically in clinical epidemiology.[3] In a seminal article that was published in 1992, the Evidence-Based Medicine Working Group argued that using evidence to inform and guide practice represented a new way of working.[4] This has been borne out subsequently in the embedding of evidence-based practice in clinical care and education, not only in medicine but also in the other healthcare professions. Indeed evidence-based practice now extends well beyond healthcare to other professional groups, such as teachers. Often there has been an emphasis on randomised controlled trials as the 'gold standard' of evidence, although as evidence-based practice has matured, a broader spectrum of research evidence has been acknowledged as being potentially valuable.[5] For example, in nursing and midwifery there is a growing body of qualitative research evidence available in a wide range of specialties, including breastfeeding. Such research can be useful to practitioners as evidence, but can often be difficult to appraise and assess, as qualitative research tends to be context-specific, and needs to be closely scrutinised for its transferability to other settings, be they geographical, clinical, cultural or social.

An evidence-based approach to professional practice is now fully embedded in the healthcare professions, with regulatory bodies mandating the professions under their jurisdiction to comply with evidence-based practice. For example, the Nursing and Midwifery Council (NMC), in its *Code: standards of conduct, performance and ethics for nurses and midwives*, stipulates that nurses and midwives should make use of the best evidence they are able to access.[1]

Evidence-based practice is thus an integral part of professional practice, and healthcare professionals are expected to adopt an evidence-based approach to their practice, but this requirement presupposes a level of knowledge and understanding of what constitutes evidence, how it can be interpreted, whether it is relevant to the particular practice situation, and how to apply it in practice. For healthcare professionals working in breastfeeding this is particularly pertinent in relation to their role as information givers, supporting women to make informed choices about feeding their infants.

The Centre for Evidence-Based Medicine outlines the five steps involved in evidence-based practice (www.cebm.net/index.aspx?o=1914). These require practitioners to develop different skills related to literature retrieval, critique of research studies and applicability to practice. The five steps are outlined in Box 6.1.

Box 6.1: The five steps involved in evidence-based practice (reproduced with permission of the Centre for Evidence-Based Medicine)

1. **Asking focused questions:** translation of uncertainty into an answerable question.
2. **Finding the evidence:** systematic retrieval of the best evidence available.
3. **Critical appraisal:** testing the evidence for validity, clinical relevance and applicability.
4. **Making a decision:** application of the results in practice.
5. **Evaluating performance:** auditing evidence-based decisions.

These steps are each in their own right potentially time-consuming and complex. Furthermore, there are recognised barriers to evidence-based practice which need to be considered and which are relevant to professionals who are promoting and supporting breastfeeding. For example, in a study of 458 nurses working in an academic medical centre, it was found that the most significant barriers to evidence-based practice were organisational factors related to insufficient time and lack of autonomy and support to implement change. Other barriers were related to finding and interpreting the literature itself.[6]

The issues described above show that although evidence-based practice is an important part of the healthcare professional's role, becoming proficient in evidence-based practice requires specific competencies, and can be affected by the organisational structure in which the healthcare professional is working. Becoming a confident and competent evidence-based practitioner requires active development of the associated skills over time. In the next section of this chapter we shall discuss some issues related to evidence-based practice which are specific to the promotion and support of breastfeeding.

IDENTIFYING AND ANALYSING CURRENT AREAS OF RESEARCH

In Chapter 1 we discussed the growing awareness of breastfeeding as an international issue, and there is a need to carry out breastfeeding research not just at local or national levels, but with international policies and comparisons in mind. A report by Protheroe *et al.* suggested that breastfeeding studies (whether locally, nationally or internationally based) should allow comparisons to be made between countries and similar social groupings.[7] This report also made recommendations on conducting research to support the transferability of results, and to facilitate the integration of research into practice. Four issues that emerged from the report are particularly relevant to evidence-based practice.

➤ There need to be clear, universally accepted definitions for breastfeeding.
➤ Research studies should be of an appropriate size, and a suitable research design should be used.
➤ Qualitative methods can help to identify women's views.
➤ Data collection methods should be applied that allow comparison of results across regions.[8]

Guidelines and reviews, such as those developed by Renfrew *et al.* and Protheroe *et al.*, can be used to help to evaluate local practices and conventions and to make an assessment of national and international research on breastfeeding.[9,10]

Just as there are practice issues which will vary between local areas and different countries, so research themes in breastfeeding vary from one area to another, and from one country to another. For example, breastfeeding and HIV/AIDS is an issue of international importance, but it is most relevant in countries with a high incidence of HIV/AIDS among women of childbearing age in the population.

Although research studies are a valuable source of evidence to aid policy making and clinical decision making, research also performs a useful function in identifying gaps in knowledge (i.e. those areas where more research is needed). Because breastfeeding is often a highly political issue (*see* Chapter 1), it is imperative that healthcare professionals have a thorough understanding not only of what is known, but also of where knowledge is lacking.

A range of research themes have been identified for which additional research studies are needed, as summarised in Box 6.2.[11]

Box 6.2: Breastfeeding themes that require additional research

- Effectiveness of breastfeeding information and timing of health promotion. activities, including the involvement of partners in breastfeeding promotion.
- Studies linked to low-income groups and socially disadvantaged women.
- Self-help strategies.
- Comparative studies between breastfeeding and bottle feeding.
- Effectiveness of training programmes for healthcare professionals, including specialist courses.

- Cultural and ethnic minority research, including comparative studies.
- Support for initiation of breastfeeding (one-to-one vs. group methods).
- Cost-effectiveness of interventions.
- Evaluation of public acceptability of and support for breastfeeding, including the effectiveness of media campaigns.
- Value of different approaches to peer support.
- Use of multi-faceted interventions to promote and support breastfeeding.
- Impact of policy initiatives on breastfeeding rates.

In a landmark review conducted in 2005, public health interventions and their effectiveness in supporting breastfeeding were evaluated.[12] This review identified significant gaps in the literature and recommended that further research and information are required about a range of issues related to public health interventions, as shown in Box 6.3.

Box 6.3: Breastfeeding and public health interventions: areas for additional research[13]

- Clinical problems encountered by mothers when breastfeeding, including insufficient milk, sore nipples and engorgement.
- Problems encountered by babies during initiation and continuation of breastfeeding.
- Practice in relation to mothers and babies with specific health needs.
- Public policy on breastfeeding.
- The reasons why some women choose to discontinue breastfeeding.
- Appropriate interventions that promote and sustain breastfeeding, including the reasons why some interventions are particularly effective but others are not.
- The views of women.
- The views of healthcare professionals involved in supporting infant feeding.
- Targeting mothers who live in the most disadvantaged communities, and the identified need for effective interventions to support breastfeeding in areas where there is social deprivation.

It can be seen that for those who are interested in undertaking research, there are still wide gaps in knowledge relating to the promotion, initiation and support of breastfeeding. For healthcare professionals who are assessing the existing evidence, it is also important to recognise and acknowledge the areas and issues for which the evidence is inadequate or inconclusive.

CONSISTENCY OF TERMINOLOGY AND INFORMATION TRANSFER
Standardising terminology

In breastfeeding, as in many other healthcare specialties, interpretation of the evidence is made more difficult when terminology is not defined and used consistently. Traditionally, the terms that have been used to define breastfeeding in the literature have been ambiguous, leading to inconsistencies in data reporting and confusion in establishing clear evidence for practice.[14] The need for global transparency, consistency and consensus on common definitions and terms used to inform practices in breastfeeding has emerged as a consistent theme in reviews of the evidence.[15-17] Clarification of definitions and terms has the potential to improve information giving for healthcare professionals and lay people, as well as to assist in the translation of knowledge and research evidence into practice, and to facilitate more effective decision-making practices.

Consensus about language use is therefore fundamental to accurate and rigorous interpretation of research results, communication of evidence and sharing of knowledge between the healthcare professional and the women for whom they care, as well as across cultural and geographical boundaries. In the late 1980s the Inter-Agency Group for Action on Breastfeeding was set up to identify and agree standard terms to reflect different types of breastfeeding behaviour. This group acknowledged that the term 'breastfeeding' alone was insufficient to describe the numerous types of breastfeeding behaviour, and it sought to standardise the terminology for breastfeeding behaviour. The following five principles reflect the focus of the Inter-Agency Group work.[18]

➤ Acknowledge that the term 'breastfeeding' alone is insufficient to describe the numerous types of breastfeeding behaviour.
➤ Distinguish between full and partial breastfeeding.
➤ Subdivide full breastfeeding into categories of exclusive and almost-exclusive breastfeeding.
➤ Differentiate between levels of partial breastfeeding.
➤ Recognise that token breastfeeding has little or no nutritional impact.

The resulting framework could be used by researchers and agencies globally to define breastfeeding in a way that supported clarity and transparency in practice, education and research. The framework standardised terminology and distinguished between full and partial breastfeeding, further subdividing full breastfeeding into categories of exclusive and almost exclusive breastfeeding. Partial and token breastfeeding were also recognised as definitions in their own right.[19] This framework was useful for healthcare professionals when reviewing the literature and research evidence and when analysing breastfeeding practices. It also represented a potentially valuable way of facilitating communication between different healthcare professionals, and between professionals and the women whom they support.

Six years later, the WHO reviewed and modified the Inter-Agency Group framework for the Global Data Bank on Breastfeeding, further refining the definitions used in practice.[20] In the 1996 revisions the previous differentiation between exclusive and almost exclusive breastfeeding is not made explicit, but the increasing number of infants receiving breast milk from a wet nurse is acknowledged. This WHO revised framework is currently the recommended guideline for terminology to be used in breastfeeding.

ELIMINATING CONFLICTING AND COMPETING ADVICE

Healthcare professionals practise as part of the healthcare team, rather than working in isolation, and mothers who hope to breastfeed or who are already breastfeeding will receive information from different members of the healthcare team. The ability to communicate clearly with other team members, as well as with the women for whom they provide care, is therefore an additional challenge in information giving and knowledge transfer. Furthermore, there is evidence to suggest that lack of advice or negative advice from healthcare professionals can be a major obstacle to successful breastfeeding.[21] This finding highlights the need for the healthcare team to take a collective and evidence-based approach to the promotion and support of breastfeeding, to help to ensure that women receive consistent and high-quality information. A review of studies that have evaluated educational interventions to promote healthy feeding of infants under 1 year of age found that success was most likely when the intervention took place over time and involved a number of contacts with the mother.[22] Such an approach necessitates collaboration and cooperation among the members of the team.

In the next section of this chapter, studies that examine issues which are directly and indirectly related to breastfeeding will be discussed. Although the issues examined in the studies are themselves relevant to practitioners working in breastfeeding, they also act as worked examples of how to evaluate evidence and focus on the third step listed in Box 6.1, namely the critical appraisal of evidence.

EXAMINING THE EVIDENCE

Five case studies that examine research themes related to breastfeeding have been chosen and analysed in order to demonstrate the types of research that are associated with breastfeeding practice and how that research has evolved over time. The discussion identifies specific issues related to each theme, and exposes the challenges and opportunities for those conducting research or disseminating research evidence.

Case 1
Dental caries: complexities and inconclusive research evidence
In 1998, a study by Palmer investigated a possible connection between breastfeeding and dental caries in the primary teeth of infants.[23] The study concluded that human milk alone does not cause dental caries, and reported that dental

caries is caused by several factors other than breast milk, such as exposure to the decay-causing bacterium *Streptococcus mutans*, which is transmitted to the infant via the parents, caregivers and others.

Then, in 2000, a review of the literature on infant dental caries was undertaken which found contradictions in the research designs used and in the way that analyses were performed, due to choices of research methods, variables and definitions.[24] The review team found apparent inconsistencies with regard to how risk factors were presented and evaluated. From this review of the literature they refuted previous research claims of a consistent and strong relationship between breastfeeding and the development of early childhood caries (ECC). Through their systematic review of the literature, Valaitis and colleagues concluded that there is no right time to stop breastfeeding with regard to prevention of ECC, and that mothers should be encouraged to breastfeed for as long as they wish.[25] They also recommended that future research in this area should:

➤ employ more rigorous research protocols
➤ use consistent definitions of ECC
➤ include data on variables for infant feeding and infant care practices (e.g. dental health practices)
➤ ideally be conducted by an inter-disciplinary team.

To support informed decision making by parents on this issue, further research appears to be needed into the relationship between ECC and breastfeeding.

The Palmer study highlights the complexity of research results and the need to interpret findings with care.[26] It also emphasises the uncertainty and inherent complexity of most research areas, which require informed consideration to tease out intricate and interwoven cause-and-effect relationships. It can also be important to acknowledge the uncertainties and the inconclusive nature of the evidence that is generated by research. This conclusion is supported by the systematic review conducted by Valaitis *et al.*, which highlighted the need for informed professionals to interpret research findings in a reliable way so that information which is communicated to the public is accurate, clear, consistent and up to date.[27] This illustrates the need for professionals to comprehend and interpret complicated and inconclusive research evidence.

Case 2
Comparing formula feeding and breastfeeding: the potentially political nature of evidence

This case study is about sociological research by Lee and Furedi, published in 2005, which examined how women experience feeding their babies, and which has been the subject of national publicity and debate in the UK.[28] It illustrates how research can be used in political and controversial ways, whether or not that was the original intention of the research.

This was a two-part study, which reported on in-depth qualitative interviews with 33 wholly or partially formula-feeding mothers and a sample of 503 mothers who participated in telephone interviews and who were either breast-feeding or formula feeding.

The controversial subject and results of this study highlight the necessity for healthcare professionals to be skilled in the interpretation of research results with regard to study design and research methods. For example, the details of recruitment, sample demographics and ethical considerations were not reported. An additional factor for consideration is that this study was funded by the Infant and Dietetic Foods Association, representing the manufacturers of specialist nutrition products. This is presently known as the British Specialist Nutrition Association.

The study examined four aspects of the use of formula, namely why women choose to bottle-feed, how women find out about formula feeding, how women perceive the information that they receive about formula feeding, and how women feel about using formula milk, including when relating to the healthcare professionals whom they encounter, other mothers and their own partners.

The results are presented in an academic report, and although the design and funding of the research can be questioned, the results are clearly set out, with assertions that are made being backed up by direct quotes from the women who were interviewed. Although the report challenges societal attitudes to bottle-feeding women, it does so within an academic framework (the full report can be accessed at www.kent.ac.uk/sspssr/staff/academic/lee/infant-formula-full.pdf).

However, when the research was reported in the media, it was introduced by the value-laden headline 'Breast may not be best after all, says professor.'[29] The article asserted that bottle-feeding women had been made to feel as if they were inferior parents, and that the dangers of adversely affecting women's belief in their abilities as a mother in this way were much more serious than any possible health risks associated with babies drinking formula. Clearly, the media is free to report research from its own particular perspective, political or otherwise, and to report only selected aspects of the research. The challenge for the healthcare professional is to be a step ahead of sensational and political reporting, and to be prepared to provide factual, unbiased information that sets aside sensational reporting. Healthcare professionals also need to take the time and opportunity to untangle any areas of misinformation, confusion and controversy.

Case 3
Peer support for breastfeeding: identifying lack of conclusive evidence and areas for further research

The concept of peer support has been of interest since the early 1990s.[30-36] The wide range of variables associated with peer support and breastfeeding (cultural, socio-economic, psychological and healthcare related) have led to contradictory and inconclusive research results. This reduces considerably the transferability of research findings to specific local practice. Randomised controlled trials are particularly difficult to undertake with regard to peer support, because of the inability to control variables. According to Britton *et al.*, the evidence on the effectiveness of peer support remains inconclusive, but enough positive evidence is available to encourage further studies and investigation.[37]

Systematic reviews can be extremely helpful in summarising evidence from current studies and providing guidance on potential research gaps (i.e. those areas where additional evidence would be beneficial). The review by Fairbank *et al.* on the effectiveness of peer support reported that peer support programmes, as stand-alone interventions for women who stated that they wished to breast-feed, were found to be effective, but they were not effective for those women who had decided to bottle-feed.[38] It was also found that peer support can be success-fully delivered as part of a multi-faceted intervention approach. For example, incorporating opportunities for women to see and talk to other women who are or have been successful in breastfeeding may be useful as part of a 'package' of support for breastfeeding.

In research areas such as peer support for breastfeeding, the multiplicity of variables can lead to bias, which may compromise the value of the evidence that is generated. For example, Dennis *et al.* found that peer support enhanced breast-feeding initiation, exclusive breastfeeding and continuation rates.[39] However, in this study the high initiation rates may have been indicative of a positive breastfeeding culture that was present at the start of the study, and that may not be present in other similar studies. This therefore introduced an element of bias to this study, which needs to be taken into consideration when interpreting the results with regard to their applicability to different healthcare cultures, and if designing new studies in this area. Bias in a research study refers to any distor-tion of the results, intentional or otherwise.[40] Most bias will be unintentional, but it can arise from many different sources, such as identification of variables, inability to control variables, wording of questionnaires or interpretation of the results. Bias must be reduced as much as possible as part of the rigour applied to the research design.

Despite the wealth of information that is available on peer review, there appears to be a dearth of studies in certain areas. For example, in a 2005 review on public health interventions to promote the duration of breastfeeding, around 55 000 citations were identified, but only 17 studies examined the needs of women from the most disadvantaged groups.[41] The Renfrew review identified the following areas to be considered when assessing research on peer review or implementing practice initiatives for peer support interventions.[42]

➤ Specific breastfeeding support from peers and professionals has been shown to be effective in increasing breastfeeding among those women who have planned to breastfeed, so long as the support is offered soon after birth.

➤ Peer support has been shown to increase exclusive breastfeeding in women from advantaged backgrounds.

➤ Peer support has not been shown to be effective in increasing breastfeeding among women from disadvantaged backgrounds.

➤ Additional postnatal support, regardless of feeding intention or practice, is unlikely to affect the duration of breastfeeding.

> There is no evidence that professionals without breastfeeding-specific training have been effective in supporting women to breastfeed.

The Renfrew review also identified the following areas of research on breastfeeding peer support that could benefit from further research and the generation of more evidence:[43]

> communities with low rates of breastfeeding initiation
> the effectiveness of lay support from within the local community
> the effectiveness of professional support
> the effectiveness of training programmes
> the cost-effectiveness of different interventions
> comparative studies across different countries
> comparative studies of major initiatives, such as the Baby-Friendly Initiative
> qualitative research to explore the perspective of breastfeeding women.

The research area of peer support is a good example of how, despite the fact that a large number of studies have been conducted, uncertainties can remain about evidence relating to benefits and outcomes. However, with such a body of research, the gaps in knowledge and the priority areas for future research topics are well understood.

Case 4
Solitary sleeping/co-sleeping and SIDS: the culturally or socially specific nature of research evidence

In many parts of the world, such as Africa, co-sleeping is the norm and may occur because of tradition and for reasons of economic necessity rather than psychological comfort. Solitary sleeping or co-sleeping behaviour is therefore closely linked to societal traditions, the prevailing values and attitudes within a society, and the individual nature of each family unit. It is therefore accepted that across different countries and cultures ideas about sleeping arrangements vary enormously, and that the majority of sleeping practices are socially and culturally led and are closely influenced by the attitudes of men as well as cultural attitudes towards birth, babies and breastfeeding.[44]

In Western societies, solitary sleeping arrangements are commonplace and may be associated with a variety of practical reasons, such as availability of space and shift work, and may also relate to values and beliefs such as fostering independence in infants and children. In comparison, Mayan mothers do not believe in separate sleeping quarters for the family, and view solitary sleeping of a baby with disapproval, regarding this practice as neglecting the essential needs of the infant.[45] A logical conclusion is therefore that sleep habits which are identified as 'normal' physiologically are socially invented, and may in fact be an adaptation to the preferred habits of parents.[46]

This variation in ideas and norms with regard to solitary and co-sleeping means that research evidence on such topics needs to be assessed with care, as the results may not be transferable to different situations.

In the early 1990s, bed sharing in the developed world was associated with concerns about sudden infant death syndrome (SIDS). These concerns were justified a decade later, when a direct relationship was reported between the prevalence of bed sharing and an increase in sudden, unexpected death in infancy.[47] However, other reputable studies continue to advocate and support bed sharing. For example, Davies suggests that the optimum progress of the infant is associated with the potential benefits of mothers co-sleeping with their babies.[48] This view is supported by research evidence from the medical anthropologist James McKenna, who speculates that co-sleeping supports the development of neurological and physiological mechanisms which underlie the arousal response.[49]

The work of McKenna demonstrates that co-sleeping mothers wake 6 to 10 times during the night to check or attend to their baby, and frequently have no recollection of this nocturnal activity. His studies also found that babies sleeping with their mothers:

➤ arouse more frequently
➤ have wake–sleep patterns which synchronise with that of the mother
➤ wake up to feed three times more often than babies who sleep apart from their mothers.

Although McKenna's research study contributes valuable evidence of the benefits of bed sharing and breastfeeding, the study requires closer scrutiny when interpreting the results. For example, the mothers in this study were of middle-class background and thus were not a representative sample of the social diversity that is generally found in any given society. Therefore there were maternal variables associated with social class, level of education and environment, which may have influenced the results of the research and reduced the generalisability, and hence the transferability, of the results.

Additional studies in this area indicate that co-sleeping patterns in breastfeeding and non-breastfeeding parents differ. In particular, breastfeeding mothers generally adopt a position where they are curled around the baby, whereas bottle-feeding couples are more likely to turn their backs on the baby.

Based on the prevailing evidence emerging from research centres, the Baby-Friendly Initiative actively promoted the principle of 'rooming in' to keep mother and baby together while the mother and baby are in hospital. The *Fabella Experience* in a large hospital in the Philippines is an example of how the Baby-Friendly guidelines on rooming in were interpreted in a particular cultural context and then applied to practice. The essence of the Fabella Experience was that baby cots were removed from postnatal wards and replaced by floor mattresses so that the mother and baby could sleep together.[50,51] Such an approach would not necessarily be acceptable or practicable in other countries or cultures, but it shows how evidence can be interpreted and transferred into practice, taking account of local needs and the norms or acceptable practices of a society.

Other studies have challenged bed sharing and identified contraindications and risks to infants from bed sharing with adult members of the family.[52,53] One study found that bed sharing is only associated with SIDS if a parent is a smoker.[54] This research generated considerable debate about the reliability of the evidence. Subsequent research refuted these findings, based on results that indicated a high risk of SIDS in young infants who were bed sharing, even if their parents did not smoke.[55] In the UK, a change in practice at national and local level has occurred. In the absence of conclusive evidence, parents are advised by government that it is not safe to bed share during the first 3 months of an infant's life, regardless of any other factors.

The lack of conclusive evidence to support either the benefits or disadvantages of co-sleeping and solitary sleeping for both baby and family can be confusing, especially given the variety of social attitudes and norms with regard to these different practices. The challenge for the healthcare professional is to provide factual information, taking account of the research evidence, while having to convey often contradictory results to women and families. Furthermore, varying traditions and norms in different societies and cultures mean that healthcare professionals need to be sensitive to different needs or expectations, particularly when working in multicultural communities.

The evidence on co-sleeping and solitary sleeping is a good example of the culturally and socially specific nature of some research evidence. It is important to be aware of this when appraising research evidence and assessing its relevance to a particular practice situation.

Case 5
Human immunodeficiency virus (HIV): applying research evidence to comply with local and national policies and legal requirements

The Global Strategy for Infant and Young Child Feeding documented the large number of babies being born annually (around 1.6 million) to women who are HIV-positive.[56] This problem is more prevalent in lower-income nations. HIV infection can be transmitted through breast milk, and may ultimately cause acquired immune deficiency syndrome (AIDS), resulting in destruction of the immune system, with the associated susceptibility to invasion by other infections, such as tuberculosis.[57] Babies born to HIV-positive mothers have their mother's antibodies to the virus in their circulation until at least 10 months of age, when the child will generate their own antibodies.[58] The HIV status of the child will not be known until this time.

The WHO advocates that all HIV-infected mothers should receive counselling and advice, including the nutritional requirements for both mother and infant, and the feeding options most suitable for their situation.[59] In developed nations this recommendation is generally given by healthcare professionals. For example, in the UK, HIV-positive mothers are counselled to use infant formula, due to the risk of transmission of the virus in breast milk and the low infant mortality rates associated with formula use.[60,61] Furthermore, any mother in the UK who is known to be HIV-positive and who chooses to breastfeed will have to undergo an enquiry under Section 47 of the Children's Act 1989, because of the risk of physical abuse to the child by breastfeeding and thus risking transmission of HIV.[62]

A Cochrane systematic review of the literature reported that the use of the antiretroviral drugs zidovudine and nevirapine appears to reduce the risk of HIV transmission from mother to child.[63] Caesarean section also appears to be a mode of infant delivery that further reduces the risk of transmission.[64] There is limited availability of these two interventions in developing countries.

Evidence from another study found that babies who were exclusively breast-fed and then changed to mixed feeding had an increased likelihood of acquiring HIV infection.[65] This was thought to be due to damage to the gut, which facilitated entry of HIV from the breast milk through to the body tissues of the infant. There is also evidence to suggest that HIV-infected mothers who breastfeed exclusively for 3 months or longer cause no greater risk of HIV infection during the first 6 months of life than the mothers of babies who are not breastfed.[66]

In the developing world, the absolute risk of HIV transmission through breastfeeding for more than 1 year, which is globally in the range 10–20% of children, needs to be balanced against the increased risk of morbidity and mortality through respiratory and gastroenteritis infections when infants are not breastfed.[67] A very different set of circumstances therefore makes the developing nations' situation more complex than that of the developed world. Different sets of issues exist in the developed and developing worlds, including geographical, social, cultural, economic and health factors. This fact serves to highlight the importance of undertaking research from a local and/or national perspective and interpreting research evidence in the context of local and/or national policies and acceptable practices.

WHO policy at the end of 2008, based on evidence to date, advised that HIV-positive women should be encouraged to breastfeed in developing countries but not in developed countries.[68] The difference in policy between the developing and developed worlds relates to economic factors, health factors, health systems and demographic data on factors such as infant mortality rates associated with the use of formula feeding for infants in developing countries. Emerging evidence suggests that we do not have a full understanding of mother-to-child transmission of HIV. The related argument for promoting free formula milk in countries where HIV infection is prevalent is therefore spurious, and this issue remains controversial. It has been suggested that 'breast is still best', even when HIV prevalence is high.[69]

The above discussion demonstrates that there are areas of research evidence relating to HIV infection and breastfeeding which are quite clear. However, the interpretation of this evidence and the practice strategies that are applied in the light of the evidence may need to differ, depending on the local or national situation. The approach to breastfeeding in HIV-positive women is a good example of this situation.

PRACTICE PERSPECTIVE: CRITIQUING RESEARCH STUDIES AND IMPLEMENTING EVIDENCE-BASED PRACTICE

These five case studies demonstrate the complex and often uncertain nature of research evidence. Healthcare professionals need to be research aware and observant of cause-and-effect relationships in their own practice context. It is possible to develop a research approach in day-to-day work through a heightened awareness of cause-and-effect relationships and through using experience of local traditions and practices to inform the critiquing of research evidence. For example, understanding of the way that family support systems can affect women's decision making or options can help to give direction on how research evidence can best be presented or applied for individual women and their own specific circumstances. It is also important to gain competence in interpreting and presenting controversial or complex evidence. Healthcare professionals are expected to provide up-to-date, objective and accurate information on relevant healthcare issues, and this requires an ability to tease out areas of conflicting evidence and to present patient information clearly and logically, while also maintaining consistency, accuracy and objectivity. This can be challenging, particularly in situations when the evidence is inconclusive or controversial.

It is accepted that research and application of evidence to practice can be an area that healthcare professionals find difficult, and that has documented barriers.[70] Even though individual practitioners may wish to apply evidence to their own practice, they may encounter institutional barriers when trying to bring this about, and this is often particularly difficult for the more junior members of a team.[71]

However, engagement with evidence-based practice is no longer an exception but is now an expectation of the healthcare professional.[72] All professionals should have access to literature, through online databases, to enable them to keep their practice current and to be aware of up-to-date evidence. Fundamental to the effective application of research evidence to practice is the need for healthcare professionals to be able to differentiate between research and opinion-based literature, and professionals also need to have the capability, time and opportunity to access and select relevant articles, which may be challenging in the context of caring for patients and clients. There is thus a need to have the competence to critically review publications, in order to identify reliable and credible findings.

Critical review of research publications therefore involves objective evaluation of research design, methods and outcomes in order to ascertain their strengths and weaknesses and their ultimate relevance to practice. The critiquing process consists of a critical appraisal of the main elements that should be clearly identified in research studies. It does not include dogmatic exposure of every mistake, but rather checking that the study is unbiased, as well as uncovering the study's strengths, weaknesses and relevance.[73] Research-based articles *broadly* follow a common format, as shown in Table 6.1. This can be used as a guide for critiquing, although it is important to be aware that formats do vary from one journal to another, and according to the type of research that has been undertaken.

TABLE 6.1: Format of published research papers

Title	Gives a clear indication of the topic covered in the paper.
Abstract	Summarises key aspects of the paper.
Introduction	'Sets the scene' for the paper, and may include background information.
Literature review	Provides a review of the relevant literature and clarifies the need for the study.
Method	Sets out the method chosen and how it was operationalised.
Results	Describes the results or findings of the study and how they were analysed.
Discussion	Analyses the research study, identifying its strengths and weaknesses, as well as its implications for practice.
Conclusion	May include key outcomes of the study and recommendations for further research.
References	The format of references will vary according to the requirements of the journal.

To assess the relative value of research studies to professional practice requires an understanding of the research process and of how to critique research articles. Frameworks are available which can help with critical appraisal of research papers. Cutcliffe and Ward have reviewed a number of such frameworks,[74] and there are others freely available online. For example, in the UK the NHS has developed a range of critiquing tools through the Critical Appraisal Skills Programme (CASP). These are specific to different types of research designs (and can be accessed online at www.phru.nhs.uk/pages/PHD/resources.htm).

Frameworks can be helpful when one is reading articles, as they assist with identifying the relevance, validity, strengths and weaknesses of a paper.

CONCLUSION

Current research evidence clearly supports the promotion of breastfeeding as the optimum form of infant nutrition.[75] However, evidence-based practice in breastfeeding is not without its challenges. Many breastfeeding-related topics require further research, while others have generated research evidence which is contradictory or inconclusive. Added to this is the multiplicity of factors involved, including cultural, social, economic, developmental and political issues, which can make breastfeeding research difficult to transfer to different situations.

Since the 1990s, the quality of breastfeeding research and evaluative studies has attracted considerable attention, much of it negative.[76-79] It is therefore important that professionals can assess for themselves the value and relevance of research studies to local and national policy, practice and service development. Developing an awareness of how to appraise research studies, coupled with an in-depth understanding of the issues and cause-and-effect relationships in the professional's local situation, can equip healthcare professionals with the skills to support and inform women and their families in a sensitive and individual way.

FURTHER READING

A summary of work by Palmer in relation to dental caries and breastfeeding can be found on his website (at www.brianpalmerdds.com/bfeed_caries.htm).

There are a number of online databases of nursing and healthcare literature which can be accessed and searched openly. These include the following:
➤ Medline: www.ncbi.nlm.nih.gov/entrez
➤ The British Nursing Index: www.bniplus.co.uk

REFERENCES

1 Nursing and Midwifery Council. *The Code: standards of conduct, performance and ethics for nurses and midwives*. London: Nursing and Midwifery Council; 2008
2 Spring B. Evidence-based practice in clinical psychology: what it is, why it matters; what you need to know. *J Clin Psychol*. 2007; **63**: 611–31.
3 Heller R, Page J. A population perspective to evidence-based medicine: 'evidence for population health.' *J Epidemiol Community Health*. 2002; **56**: 45–7.
4 Evidence-Based Medicine Working Group. A new approach to teaching the practice of medicine. *JAMA*. 1992; **268**: 2420–5.
5 DiCenso A, Cullum N, Ciliska D. Implementing evidence-based nursing: some misconceptions. *Evid Base Nurs*. 1998; **1**: 38–9.
6 Brown CE, Wickline MA, Ecoff L *et al*. Nursing practice, knowledge, attitudes and perceived barriers to evidence-based practice at an academic medical center. *J Adv Nurs*. 2009; **65**: 371–81.
7 Protheroe L, Dyson L, Renfrew M. *The Effectiveness of Public Health Interventions to Promote the Initiation of Breastfeeding*. Evidence Briefing. London: Health Development Agency; 2003.
8 Ibid.
9 Renfrew MJ, Dyson L, Wallace L *et al*. *The Effectiveness of Public Health Interventions to Promote the Duration of Breastfeeding: systematic review*. London: National Institute for Health and Clinical Excellence; 2005. www.nice.org.uk/page.aspx?o=511622 (accessed 5 October 2009).
10 Protheroe L, Dyson L, Renfrew M, op. cit.
11 Ibid.
12 Renfrew MJ, Dyson L, Wallace L *et al*., op. cit.
13 Ibid.
14 Protheroe L, Dyson L, Renfrew M, op. cit.
15 Tedstone A, Dunce N, Aviles M *et al*. *Effectiveness of Interventions to Promote Healthy*

Feeding of Infants under One Year of Age: review. London: Health Education Authority; 1998. www.nice.org.uk/page.aspx?o=501963 (accessed 5 October 2009).

16 Fairbank L, O'Meara S, Renfrew MJ *et al.* A systematic review to evaluate the effectiveness of interventions to promote the initiation of breastfeeding. *Health Technol Assess.* 2000; **4**: 1–171.

17 Renfrew MJ, Dyson L, Wallace L *et al.*, op. cit.

18 Labbok MH, Krasovec K. Towards consistency in breastfeeding definitions. *Stud Fam Plann.* 1990; **21**: 226–30.

19 Ibid.

20 World Health Organization. *WHO Global Data Bank on Breastfeeding.* Geneva: World Health Organization; 1996.

21 Johnston M, Esposito N. Barriers and facilitators for breastfeeding among working women in the United States. *J Obstet Gynecol Neonatal Nurs.* 2007; **36**: 9–20.

22 Tedstone A, Dunce N, Aviles M *et al.*, op. cit.

23 Palmer B. The influence of breastfeeding on the development of the oral cavity: a commentary. *J Hum Lact.* 1998; **14**: 93–8.

24 Valaitis R, Hesch R, Passarelli C *et al.* A systematic review of the relationship between breastfeeding and early childhood caries. *Can J Public Health.* 2000; **91**: 411–17.

25 Ibid.

26 Palmer B, op. cit.

27 Valaitis R, Hesch R, Passarelli C *et al.*, op. cit.

28 Lee E, Furedi F. *Mothers' Experience of, and Attitudes to, using Infant Formula in the Early Months.* 2005. www.kent.ac.uk/sspssr/staff/academic/lee/infant-formula-full.pdf (accessed 3 November 2009).

29 Frean A. Breast may not be best after all, says professor. *The Times*, 5 July 2005.

30 Guigliani E, Caiaffa W, Vogelhut J *et al.* Effect of breastfeeding support from different sources on mothers' decisions to breastfeed. *J Hum Lact.* 1994; **10**: 157–61.

31 Humphreys AS, Thompson NJ, Miner KR. Intention to breastfeed in low-income pregnant women: the role of social support and previous experience. *Birth.* 1998; **25**: 169–74.

32 Schafer E, Vogel MK, Viegas S *et al.* Volunteer peer counsellors increase breastfeeding duration among rural low-income women. *Birth.* 1998; **25**: 101–6.

33 Pugh LC, Milligan RA, Brown LP. The breastfeeding support team for low-income, predominantly minority women: a pilot intervention study. *Health Care Women Int.* 2001; **22**: 501–15.

34 Dennis C, Hodnett E, Gallop R *et al.* The effect of peer support on breastfeeding duration among primiparous women: a randomized controlled trial. *Can Med Assoc J.* 2002; **166**: 21–8.

35 Protheroe L, Dyson L, Renfrew M. *The Effectiveness of Public Health Interventions to Promote the Initiation of Breastfeeding.* Evidence Briefing. London: Health Development Agency; 2003.

36 Graffy J, Taylor J, Williams A *et al.* Randomised controlled trial of support from volunteer counsellors for mothers considering breastfeeding. *BMJ.* 2004; **328**: 26–9.

37 Britton C, McCormick F, Renfrew MJ *et al.* Support for breastfeeding mothers. *Cochrane Database Syst Rev.* 2007; **1**: CD001141.

38 Fairbank L, Woolridge M, O'Meara S *et al.*, op. cit.

39 Dennis C, Hodnett E, Gallop R *et al.*, op. cit.

40 Gillis A, Jackson W. *Research for Nurses: methods and interpretation.* Philadelphia, PA: F.A. Davis Company; 2002.

41 Renfrew MJ, Dyson L, Wallace L *et al.*, op. cit.

42 Ibid.

43 Ibid.

44 Odent M. The unknown human infant. *J Hum Lact.* 1990; **6**: 6–8.

45 Morelli GA, Rogaff B, Oppenheim D *et al.* Cultural variation in infants' sleeping arrangements: questions of independence. *Dev Psychol.* 1992; **28**: 604–13.

46 Odent M, op. cit.

47 Kemp JS, Unger B, Wilkins D *et al.* Unsafe sleep practices and an analysis of bed-sharing among infants dying suddenly and unexpectedly: results of a four-year, population-based, death-scene investigation study of sudden infant death syndrome and related deaths. *Pediatrics.* 2000; **106**: 41–8.

48 Davies L. Babies co-sleeping with parents. *Midwives.* 1995; **108**: 384–6.

49 McKenna J, Mosko S, Richard C *et al.* Experimental studies of infant–parent co-sleeping: mutual physiological and behavioral influences and their relevance to SIDS (sudden infant death syndrome). *Early Hum Dev.* 1994; **38**: 187–201.

50 Ball HL, Hooker E, Kelly PJ. Where will baby sleep? Attitudes and practices of new and experienced parents regarding co-sleeping with their newborn infants. *Am Anthropol.* 1999; **101**: 143–51.

51 Blair PS, Fleming PJ, Smith IJ *et al.* Babies sleeping with parents: case–control study of factors influencing the risk of the sudden infant death syndrome. *BMJ.* 1999; **319**: 1457–62.

52 Carpenter RG, Irgens LM, Blair PS *et al.* Sudden unexplained infant death in 20 regions in Europe: a case–control study. *Lancet.* 2004; **363**: 185–91.

53 Tappin D, Ecob R, Brooke H. Bedsharing, roomsharing, and sudden infant death syndrome in Scotland: a case–control study. *J Pediatr.* 2005; **147**: 32–7.

54 Carpenter RG, Irgens LM, Blair PS *et al.*, op. cit.

55 Tappin D, Ecob R, Brooke H, op. cit.

56 World Health Organization. *Global Strategy for Infant and Young Child Feeding.* Geneva: World Health Organization; 2003. http://whqlibdoc.who.int/publications/ 2003/9241562218.pdf (accessed 3 November 2009).

57 Ziegler JB, Cooper DA, Johnson RO *et al.* Postnatal transmission of AIDS-associated retrovirus from mother to infant. *Lancet.* 1985; **2**: 981.

58 Wall A. Advising HIV-positive mothers. *Pract Nurs.* 2004; **15**: 44–6.

59 World Health Organization, op. cit.

60 Wall A, op. cit.

61 Gartner LM, Morton J, Lawrence RA *et al.*; American Academy of Pediatrics Section on Breastfeeding. Breastfeeding and the use of human milk. *Pediatrics.* 2005; **115**: 496–506.

62 Wall A, op. cit.

63 Brocklehurst P. Interventions for reducing the risk of mother-to-child transmission of HIV infection. *Cochrane Database Syst Rev.* 2002; **1**: CD000102.

64 Ibid.

65 Coutsoudis A, Pillay K, Spooner E *et al.* Influence of infant feeding patterns on early mother-to-child transmission of HIV in Durban, South Africa: a prospective cohort study. *Lancet.* 1999; **354**: 471–6.

66 Ibid.

67 World Health Organization, op. cit.

68 Coutsoudis A, Coovadia H, Wilfert C. *HIV, Infant Feeding and More Perils for Poor People: new WHO guidelines encourage review of formula milk policies.* 2008. www.scielosp.org/scielo.php?script=sci_arttext&pid=S0042-96862008000300014&lng=en &nrm=iso (accessed 6 November 2009).

69 Dobson R. Breast is still best even when HIV prevalence is high, experts say. *BMJ.* 2002; **324:** 1474.

70 Gerrish K, Ashworth P, Lacey A *et al.* Developing evidence-based practice: experiences of senior and junior clinical nurses. *J Adv Nurs.* 2008; **62:** 62–73.

71 Ibid.

72 Nursing and Midwifery Council, op. cit.

73 Polit DF, Hungler BP. *Essentials of Nursing Research: methods, appraisal and utilization,* 5th edn. Philadelphia, PA: Lippincott; 2001.

74 Cutcliffe J, Ward M. *Critiquing Nursing Research.* London: Quay Books; 2007.

75 Britton C, McCormick F, Renfrew MJ *et al.,* op. cit.

76 Serwint JR, Wilson ME, Vogelhut JW *et al.* A randomized controlled trial of prenatal pediatric visits for urban, low-income families. *Pediatrics.* 1996; **98:** 1069–75.

77 Loh NR, Kelleher CC, Long S *et al.* Can we increase breastfeeding rates? *Ir Med J.* 1997; **90:** 100–1.

78 Coombs DW, Reynolds K, Joyner G *et al.* A self-help program to increase breastfeeding among low-income women. *J Nutr Educ.* 1998; **30:** 203–9.

79 Howard C, Howard F, Lawrence R *et al.* Office prenatal formula advertising and its effect on breastfeeding patterns. *Obstet Gynecol.* 2000; **95:** 296–303.

Concluding remarks

This book addresses a wide range of issues in breastfeeding that are of contemporary interest and relevance in both the developed and developing worlds. Written primarily for healthcare professionals, the book is also expected to attract the interest of members of the general public who have an interest in breastfeeding and a wish to influence the development of related policies, practices and healthcare services in their local area.

The first chapter selected the formulation of global, national and local policy from the 1980s onward as a logical starting point for the book, and as a foundation for subsequent chapters to explore an extensive range of relevant and contemporary issues related to breastfeeding. Chapter 1 confirmed that 'best practice' over the last three decades has been driven and directed by the development of global and national directives, clearly identified standards of practice and a growing body of research evidence. In this respect, this first chapter introduces the possibility of an identifiable policy and practice dynamic (*see* Figure A), which can be used as a barometer to measure, inform, enhance or develop local practice standards and services to promote, protect and support breastfeeding.

The strong focus of the book on breastfeeding practice is aided by the use of short vignettes taken from real-life experiences. Each chapter has addressed different perspectives on breastfeeding and demonstrated the inherent complexity and challenges that this topic commands, including the relatively high degree of professional and public interest and the correspondingly low rate of women initiating breastfeeding and continuing to breastfeed for 6 months or more. In this respect, the book can also inform, enhance and contribute to the contemporary debate on breastfeeding.

It is clear that all those involved today in protecting, promoting and supporting breastfeeding are committed to sustained and continuous effort and, critically, that they are aware of what has still to be accomplished, and where the focus of effort should be. This effort is likely to translate into further refinements and strengthening of the existing foundation of breastfeeding policy and practice, including listening more attentively to the views of women on breastfeeding

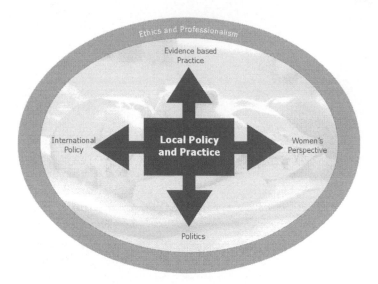

FIGURE A: Local policy and practice.

services. The general message from the leaders of this powerful and important movement is that much work has still to be done. It is the authors' hope that this book will contribute in some way towards sustaining professional effort in the twenty-first century.

LOOKING TO THE FUTURE

In November 2009, Dr Mark Cregan announced the discovery of stem cells in breast milk. The potential of this finding was generally well received, together with a note of caution to the optimists. The hope is that further research will be undertaken on a range of issues related to breast milk and breastfeeding, thereby increasing the evidence base for practice and policy, and opening the door further to increased research opportunities. At a time when global compliance with the WHO recommendation of exclusive breastfeeding until 6 months of age is low (in the UK only one-third of babies are breastfed exclusively at 1 week, and this number drops to one-fifth at 6 weeks, with only 3% of babies being exclusively breastfed at 6 months), it is hoped that further research evidence on the benefits of breast milk and breastfeeding will have a positive impact on attitudes and practices and encourage more women to breastfeed, and to breastfeed for longer.[1]

REFERENCE

1 Mesure S. Stem cells could be the secret reason why breast is best. *The Independent on Sunday*, 22 November 2009.

Further reading

The links below provide supplementary reading on a range of issues related to infants and breastfeeding. The links are all directed to WHO web pages, most of which contain official WHO reports and documentation that can be downloaded.

General

Global Strategy for Infant and Young Child Feeding:
www.who.int/entity/child_adolescent_health/topics/prevention_care/child/nutrition/global/

In February 2003 a meeting was held in Geneva to discuss the implementation of the *Global Strategy for Infant and Young Child Feeding*, and the following document is a report of that meeting, including conclusions and recommendations:
www.who.int/child_adolescent_health/documents/924159120X/en/index.html

Related to the *Global Strategy for Infant and Young Child Feeding*, the following document contains a tool for assessing national practices, policies and programmes:
www.who.int/child_adolescent_health/documents/9241562544/en/index.html

In 2007, the WHO published a planning document, aimed at supporting national implementation of the *Global Strategy for Infant and Young Child Feeding*:
www.who.int/child_adolescent_health/documents/9789241595193/en/index.html

The following WHO document provides information on community-based strategies for breastfeeding promotion and support in developing countries:
www.who.int/child_adolescent_health/documents/9241591218/en/index.html

The following document has compiled evidence to support the Ten Steps to Successful Breastfeeding:
www.who.int/child_adolescent_health/documents/9241591544/en/index.html

The following report considers the nutrient adequacy of exclusive breastfeeding for the term infant during the first 6 months of life:
www.who.int/child_adolescent_health/documents/9241562110/en/index.html

The following document contains a systematic review of the optimal feeding for low-birthweight infants:
www.who.int/child_adolescent_health/documents/9241595094/en/index.html

In 1981, the International Code of Marketing of Breast-Milk Substitutes was devised, and the following WHO publication from 2006 (updated in 2008) answers some frequently asked questions:
www.who.int/child_adolescent_health/documents/9241594292/en/index.html

The first of the following two reports is from an expert consultation on the optimal duration of exclusive breastfeeding. The second report is a systematic review of the evidence on the optimal duration of exclusive breastfeeding:
www.who.int/child_adolescent_health/documents/nhd_01_09/en/index.html
www.who.int/child_adolescent_health/documents/nhd_01_08/en/index.html

Complementary feeding

The following WHO document is a report summarising the guiding principles for complementary feeding of breastfed children: www.who.int/child_adolescent_health/documents/924154614X/en/index.html

The following discussion paper was commissioned by the WHO in 2003 to identify indicators and research priorities associated with complementary feeding:
www.who.int/child_adolescent_health/documents/discussion_146/en/index.html

HIV and infant feeding

In 2004 the WHO and UNICEF issued the following joint statement on HIV and infant feeding:
www.who.int/child_adolescent_health/documents/hiv_if_who_unicef/en/index.html

The following information on breastfeeding and replacement feeding practices in the context of mother-to-child transmission of HIV gives details of an assessment tool for use in research, as well as guidance on how to use the tool:
www.who.int/child_adolescent_health/documents/cah_01_21/en/index.html

The following document provides a framework for priority action in relation to HIV and infant feeding:
www.who.int/child_adolescent_health/documents/9241590777/en/index.html

Also in relation to HIV and infant feeding, the following WHO document provides guidelines for decision makers:
www.who.int/child_adolescent_health/documents/9241591226/en/index.html

The following guide about HIV and infant feeding, also published by the WHO, is intended for healthcare managers and supervisors:
www.who.int/child_adolescent_health/documents/9241591234/en/index.html

In relation to HIV and infant feeding, the following set of slides was devised to enable UN staff to present up-to-date information on HIV and infant feeding to partners:
www.who.int/child_adolescent_health/documents/hiv_if_slide_set/en/index.html

Published in 2007, the following document is a report of a technical consultation held on behalf of the Inter-Agency Task Team (IATT) on prevention of HIV infections in pregnant women, mothers and their infants (held in Geneva, Switzerland, on 25–27 October 2006):
www.who.int/child_adolescent_health/documents/9789241595971/en/index.html

HIV and Infant Feeding: Update (2007)
In 2007, the WHO published the following update report on current evidence on breastfeeding and HIV:
www.who.int/child_adolescent_health/documents/9789241596596/en/index.html

The following discussion paper considers home-modified animal milk for replacement feeding in relation to HIV and infant feeding:
www.who.int/child_adolescent_health/documents/a91064/en/index.html

The following document focuses on research into breastfeeding and HIV, and explores the use of formative research to adapt global recommendations on HIV and infant feeding to the local context:
www.who.int/child_adolescent_health/documents/9241591366/en/index.html

Health issues and breastfeeding

The following systematic review and meta-analysis conducted by the WHO and the University of Pelotas, Brazil, reviewed the evidence relating to breastfeeding and a range of health conditions, such as diabetes and blood pressure:

www.who.int/child_adolescent_health/documents/9241595230/en/index.html

The following document outlines the causes and management of mastitis:
www.who.int/child_adolescent_health/documents/fch_cah_00_13/en/index.html

Index